Weight Control

Weight Control

The current perspective

Edited by

Richard Cottrell

Director
The Sugar Bureau
London

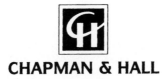

CHAPMAN & HALL

London · Glasgow · Weinheim · New York · Tokyo · Melbourne · Madras

Published by Chapman & Hall, 2–6 Boundary Row, London SE1 8HN, UK

Chapman & Hall, 2–6 Boundary Row, London SE1 8HN, UK

Blackie Academic & Professional, Wester Cleddens Road, Bishopbriggs, Glasgow G64 2NZ, UK

Chapman & Hall GmbH, Pappelallee 3, 69469 Weinheim, Germany

Chapman & Hall USA, 115 Fifth Avenue, New York, NY 10003, USA

Chapman & Hall Japan, ITP-Japan, Kyowa Building, 3F, 2-2-1 Hirakawacho, Chiyoda-ku, Tokyo 102, Japan

Chapman & Hall Australia, 102 Dodds Street, South Melbourne, Victoria 3205, Australia

Chapman & Hall India, R. Seshadri, 32 Second Main Road, CIT East, Madras 600 035, India

First edition 1995

© 1995 Chapman & Hall

Typeset in 10/12pt Palatino
Printed in Great Britain at Hartnolls Ltd, Bodmin, Cornwall

ISBN 0 412 73600 4

A catalogue record for this book is available from the British Library

Library of Congress Catalog Card Number: 95-71085

♾ Printed on permanent acid-free text paper, manufactured in accordance with ANSI/NISO Z39.48-1992 (Permanence of Paper).

Contents

Preface

The mechanisms controlling body weight or, to be more specific, that component of body mass that consists of adipose tissue is an active area of scientific research. Two stimuli can be discerned that give a sense of urgency to this research.

The first is the data, from many sources, confirming an inexorable upward trend in the prevalence of overweight and obesity in developed countries. The picture in the emerging nations is unclear because of both a lack of appropriate survey data and the continued scourge of under-nourishment among their poor. It is likely, however, that, throughout the world, wherever disposable income and food availability are high, obesity and overweight will be a continuing and increasing problem.

The second driving force among researchers is the realization that, to date, there has been little success in either stemming the tide of individuals experiencing excessive adiposity or enabling them to recover a more desirable body weight and composition.

Such are the problems. But significant progress in research into the origins and treatment of this condition is being made, and in recent years has been brisk. Technical advances (such as the ability to measure total energy expenditure in free-living individuals with good reliability), new and imaginative thinking and a determination not to be satisfied with hypotheses until they have been thoroughly challenged by experiment have yielded significant advances.

A clearer understanding of the aetiology of obesity has emerged; better approaches to treatment and prevention are being devised; better medical management of obese patients seems to have improved their morbidity and mortality risks. Progress has been impressive, but there is clearly much more to be done.

This book outlines the current state of progress and provides a number of pointers to future research. All those with an interest in the field should find it valuable. If it sparks the imagination of anyone in the field to unravel a single one of the remaining problems, I, for one, will consider its publication worthwhile.

R. C. Cottrell
London
June 1995

Acknowledgements

Thanks are due to Ministry of Health Portugal; University of Porto; Porto School of Nutrition; Comité Europeen des Fabricants de Sucre; Associacão los Refinadores le Açúcar Portugueses.

Particular mention should be made of those who have laboured on various aspects of the production of the manuscripts, especially Miss J. Leach in London and Mr G. Somerville in Brussels.

The patience and co-operation of the contributors during the editing process has eased the inevitable effort considerably and is gratefully acknowledged.

Contributors

Arne Astrup, Research Department of Human Nutrition, The Royal Veterinary and Agricultural University, Rolighedsvej 25, DK-1958 Frederiksberg C, Copenhagen, Denmark

France Bellisle, Service de Diabétologie, Hotel-Dieu, 1, Place du Parvis Notre Dame, 75181 Paris, Cedex 04, France

Michael Berger, Klinik für Stoffwechselkrankheiten und Ernährung, WHO Collaborating Centre for Diabetes, Heinrich Heine Universität Düsseldorf, Moorenstrasse 5, D-40225, Düsseldorf, Germany

Xavier Formiguera, Unidad Transtornos de la Alimentacion, Hospital Universitari Tries i Pujol, Ctra. Canyet s/n, 08015 Badalona, Spain

Susan A. Jebb, Dunn Clinical Nutrition Centre, Hills Road, Cambridge CB2 2DH, UK

Lauren Lissner, Departments of Primary Health Care and Internal Medicine, University of Göteborg, Sahlgren's Hospital, S-413 45 Göteborg, Sweden

Andrew Prentice, Dunn Clinical Nutrition Centre, Hills Road, Cambridge CB2 2DH, UK

Volker Pudel, Universität Göttingen, Zentrum 16: Psychologische Medizin, Ernährungspsychologische Forschungsstelle, Von-Siebold-Str 5, 37075 Göttingen, Germany

Anne Raben, Research Department of Human Nutrition, The Royal Veterinary and Agricultural University, Rolighedsvej, DK-1958 Frederiksberg C, Copenhagen, Denmark

Stephen Rössner, Obesity Unit, Norrbacka plan 3, Karolinska Sjukhuset, S-171 76 Stockholm, Sweden

Annebeth R. Skov, Research Department of Human Nutrition, The Royal Veterinary and Agricultural University, Rolighedsvej, DK-1958 Frederiksberg C, Copenhagen, Denmark

Claudia Sørensen, Research Department of Human Nutrition, The Royal Veterinary and Agricultural University, Rolighedsvej, DK-1958 Frederiksberg C, Copenhagen, Denmark

Søren Toubro, Research Department of Human Nutrition, The Royal Veterinary and Agricultural University, Rolighedsvej, DK-1958 Frederiksberg C, Copenhagen, Denmark

CHAPTER 1

Disease risks of obesity

Michael Berger

INTRODUCTION

The close association of obesity with increased overall mortality, cardio-vascular mortality and morbidity of various causes has become a dogma of medicine. Much of the reasoning behind this dogma is based on the North American Life Insurance Companies' data, which were published in the comprehensive Build and Blood Pressure Study in 1959 (Metropolitan Life Insurance Company, 1959). From these data, ideal body weight standards were calculated as predictors for an individual's optimal longevity. In fact, these standards have profoundly influenced the thinking and decision-making in medicine, public health and in our societies for decades. The actual evidence for these policies on the definition and evaluation of overweight and obesity as predictors and risk factors of morbidity and excess mortality will be reviewed in detail.

One often quoted example of the link between obesity and disease is the apparent close association between overweight and type II diabetes mellitus. The biometrical and pathophysiological relationship between these two conditions and the over-riding influence of genetic factors will be scrutinized by referral to various sets of original data.

Epidemiological evidence in support of obesity-associated excess mortality will be presented in relation to the degree of overweight; these data result in a challenge to the widely accepted definitions of normal weight, overweight and gross and morbid obesity. Data from the Düsseldorf Obesity Mortality Study on the mortality of a cohort of almost 5000 obese patients recruited between 1960 and 1983 are presented against standard mortality rates of the general population. These data suggest that the mortality risk, even of gross obesity [body mass index (BMI) between 30 and

Weight Control
Edited by Richard Cottrell.
Published in 1995 by Chapman & Hall, London. ISBN 0 412 73600 4

41 kg m^{-2}], appears substantially lower than is generally assumed.

The substantial increase in prevalence rates for obesity in the USA over the past three decades is discussed in contrast to the reported decrease in cardiovascular mortality.

Obesity-related risks for morbidity and mortality have too often been looked upon rather superficially in the past; detailed analyses of statistical, biometric and pathophysiological relationships between excess weight and disease risks are required before sweeping statements in the public health sector are justified.

THE FALLACY OF IDEAL BODY WEIGHT STANDARDS

Obesity is considered to be a high-priority public health problem in industrialized societies. Very few conditions or disease states have attracted so much public attention. Both the public and the medical community generally assume that a reduction in the prevalence rates for obesity will result in dramatic improvements in the population's morbidity and mortality. As a consequence, costly and sometimes even hazardous programmes have been devised to treat or to prevent obesity. While there is little doubt that serious impairment of health and well-being is caused by gross obesity, it has become quite apparent that many of the currently popular attempts to reduce more moderate degrees of overweight are not backed up by appropriate scientific or clinical evidence. In fact, the result of most public and commercial anti-obesity campaigns has been that a great many people who are, at worst, somewhat overweight are preoccupied by their weight while most really obese people are largely unimpressed. So far, very few efforts have differentiated between overweight people who want to lose weight for social or aesthetic reasons and those who really should lose weight because their obesity represents a substantial risk to their health and life expectancy. Lack of knowledge of the actual consequences and risks of obesity appears to be the main reason for this disturbing confusion. Clear-cut answers are needed to the questions 'What is obesity?' and 'Under what circumstances are therapeutic measures medically indicated to reduce obesity?'.

Until the late 1970s, at least in Germany, the dogma of the ideal body weight, derived from the Build and Blood Pressure Study of North American Life Insurance Companies, was generally accepted by the medical community and the general public alike: based upon height (and type of body frame), for every person one could calculate a precise body weight level that was associated with optimal life expectancy (Metropolitan Life Insurance Company, 1959). Any increase in the actual body weight above the individual's ideal weight was held to reduce life expectancy. To help the population and their doctors to calculate the ideal body weight for every individual, nomograms were displayed in every medical textbook and in every physician's or hospital office and every pharmacy. In general, ideal weight standards were substantially lower than the population's average body weight. In consequence, the medical profession and public health crusaders exerted pressure on the population at large to reduce weight – and they are still doing so. Despite the dogmatic nature of this approach and the resulting massive public health campaigns over the past decades, the scientific basis for the ideal body weight dogma has always been quite dubious and average body weights of our populations are nevertheless increasing at a worrying rate.

The so-called 'ideal' weight (formerly 'desirable weight') concept was derived from the observation of a cohort of 4.9 million policy-holders of North American life insurance companies between 1934 and 1954 (Society of Actuaries, 1959, 1960). However, the extrapolation of these data to the general public has been harshly criticized on methodological grounds since the early 1960s. For a number of reasons, the cohort examined could never be accepted as representative – even of the contemporary population of the USA. Systematic problems and inaccuracies with regard to the recording of height and body weight (as well as the classification of the policy-holders' body frame) could not be excluded for a number of reasons (mainly related to the purpose of recording these data, which was not in any way a scientific one). Furthermore, recalculation of the original data did not confirm a linear increase in the mortality risk with relative body weight, as recorded at the time the life insurance contract was underwritten. Rather there was an exponential relationship between relative body weight and mortality, and a significant decrease in life expectancy was not evident until the so-called ideal body weight was exceeded by 30% (Berger and Berchtold, 1978).

During the 1970s, a number of prospective epidemiological studies on defined cohorts of initially healthy people were published that were designed to document a relationship between relative body weight and life expectancy (Berger and Berchtold, 1978; Andres, 1980; Berger *et al.*, 1980, 1983). In all of these studies there was a range of relative body weight associated with low mortality rates that was substantially above the 'ideal' body weight standards. In fact, a progress report of the actuarial data of the North American life insurance companies, as published in 1980, resulted in a much wider range of 'desirable weight' standards encompassing values previously classified as moderately obese (Society of Actuaries, 1980). Only recently, more elaborate epidemiological studies based upon prospective population cohorts have been able to document the morbidity and mortality risk associated with deviations from average body weight, both under- and overweight (Rissanen *et al.*, 1989; Isles, 1992; Lee *et al.*, 1993). Some of those observations as well as their inconsistencies may be confounded, however, by cause–effect and effect–cause relationships between overweight and social classification (Gortmaker *et al.*, 1993).

In any case, it must be pointed out that, even if there is an association between increased mortality rate and a certain degree of obesity, it has not been shown that such an obesity-associated mortality risk can be reduced if obesity is successfully treated.

Since the early 1960s we have been following a cohort of some 7000 obese people by studying (among other variables) their mortality as an endpoint. Several preliminary studies published in abstract form have surprisingly, and repeatedly, revealed that the excess mortality associated with obesity was substantially less pronounced than generally expected. In fact, in women, only a body weight in excess of a BMI of 41 kg m^{-2} conferred a statistically significant decrease in life expectancy when compared with an age-matched segment of the general population living in the same geographical area (Klesse *et al.*, 1980; Berger, 1991; Trautner *et al.*, 1994). On the basis of this ongoing study it appears evident that the mortality risk of gross obesity, at least in women, is substantially lower than expected. If one takes into account, however, that for the vast majority of these patients at least one of the so-called first-order risk factors for coronary artery disease and atherosclerosis is present, one might speculate on a modification of the risk potency of such markers in patients with gross obesity – such as the prognostic value of arterial hypertension in patients with obesity (Barrett-Connor and Khaw, 1985).

OBESITY AND DIABETES: MANY AS YET UNANSWERED QUESTIONS

A large number of diseases, conditions and handicaps have been linked with overweight. Many of these associations have remained hypothetical as to their causal nature. A very strong point has always been made with regard to the link between obesity and diabetes, best known as the 'diabetic syndrome'; more recently, it has come to include hypertension, dyslipoproteinaemia, hyperuricaemia and insulin resistance, and has been called syndrome X. No doubt, in cross-sectional prevalence studies, obesity and diabetes are closely related, as well as in incidence studies covering large population cohorts over many years. Between countries and throughout the history of a country, the prevalence of obesity and diabetes wax and wane in parallel. Innumerable papers of varying epidemiological validity have been published to document the syntropy of obesity and diabetes (Gries *et al.*, 1976; West, 1978). Despite the generally accepted evidence for a strong association between glucose intolerance and obesity, the nature of the association is not a simple one; many of its details remain obscure. We do know some facts, but there are certainly more questions to be answered (Berger *et al.*, 1978).

This rather sobering view is impressively supported by the important prospective study on the predictive value of body weight for the manifestation of overt diabetes mellitus in almost 1000 women published by O'Sullivan (1982). In so-called low-risk women (without previous gestational glucose intolerance) the 10- to 16-year incidence of diabetes mellitus was low (1.9–4.5%) without any statistically significant relationship to the women's relative body weight status. However, in the so-called high-risk women (with a history of gestational glucose intolerance, probably indicative of a genetic predisposition to diabetes) the incidence of clinically overt diabetes was 10-fold higher and, indeed, there was a highly significant association with overweight (46.7% versus 25.6% in the normal-weight group). In this study, the predictive value for the manifestation of diabetes mellitus of a history of gestational glucose intolerance appeared to be almost 10-fold greater than that of obesity. On the basis of sound epidemiological studies such as the one by O'Sullivan, the generally held view that there is an overwhelming causal role of obesity (its quantity, distribution and duration) with regard to the development of type II (non-insulin-dependent) diabetes mellitus appears to have been exaggerated.

Probably overweight and obesity do have a modulating effect on the protracted process of the development of clinically overt type II diabetes mellitus, and are thus of definitive predictive value. More important, however, are genetic factors and dispositions. This may also be reflected in the impressive prevalence of type II diabetes mellitus in elderly non-overweight individuals and the fact that long-term improvements in glucose intolerance in type II diabetes mellitus achievable by weight reduction are often disappointing, even when the patients have shown impressive compliance with diet therapy and the initial results had been quite encouraging. No doubt obesity is causally related to (peripheral) insulin resistance, which is nowadays seen as a central facet of the (diabetic) syndrome X. Any reduction in overweight will assist in improving insulin sensitivity and, hence, insulin requirements of the body. In as much as a genetically transmitted defect of insulin secretion is the basis of the pathogenesis of type II diabetes mellitus, however, overweight/obesity will at best have a modulating effect on the development of the disease. Obesity may lead to an earlier exhaustion of β-cell secretory capacities and, hence, to an earlier manifestation of a disease that would otherwise manifest itself at a later time in the life of the individual.

PRESENT PUBLIC HEALTH ISSUES ON OBESITY

While public campaigns stressing the importance of slimness (and health) and maintenance of normal (if not ideal) weight standards are becoming ever more intense, actual figures on the prevalence rates of overweight and obesity tell a different tale. Recent nationally representative data from the USA have documented that the prevalence of overweight and obesity has increased quite substantially during the past 15 years (whereas rates had been rather constant between 1960 and 1975): the mean body weight for adults increased by 3.6 kg and BMI from 25.3 to 26.3 kg m^{-2} (Kuczmarski *et al.*, 1994). In fact, a very similar increase in the prevalence of obesity has been documented for England (White *et al.*, 1993) and is most likely to have occurred in other countries of the western hemisphere. This adverse effect is lamented by public health and obesity experts alike; yet it comes at a time when cardiovascular mortality is constantly decreasing and our populations enjoy ever-increasing life expectancy.

There is one other disconcerting aspect of ongoing campaigns to reduce overweight among the general public, and that is their impact on 'healthy' individuals, in whom reduction of excessive body weight does not represent the basis for any rational treatment of chronic disease (e.g. hypertension, type II diabetes, hyperlipoproteinaemia). Impressive (although not yet satisfactorily reproduced) evidence from the Framingham study has suggested that weight cycling might confer a particular mortality risk; it might in fact be more dangerous for obese individuals to lose and regain weight in cycles (the so-called 'yo-yo' phenomenon) than to remain overweight (Lissner *et al.*, 1991). If this were true, one would have to try to make sure that an overweight individual is able to maintain a lower body weight before any weight reduction treatment is initiated. At present, there is no means of predicting the success of a weight reduction programme, let alone patients' ability to maintain any weight loss achieved.

Discussion on the use of public health campaigns to reduce overweight in our populations has recently been reopened (Garrow *et al.*, 1994) without any effective methods and lasting means of treating overweight and obesity being available at the present time. Such an open and public debate is to be welcomed; however, it ought to be distinguished from the absolute need to treat obesity in patients with a number of clearly defined conditions and diseases, such as cardiovascular risk profiles, type II diabetes and hypertension.

REFERENCES

Andres R (1980). The effect of obesity on total mortality. *International Journal of Obesity* 4: 381.

Barrett-Connor E, Khaw K-T (1985). Is hypertension more benign when associated with obesity? *Circulation* 72: 53.

Berger M (1991). Risks and risk factors of obesity. In: Oomura Y, Tarui S, Inoue S, Shimazu T (eds) *Progress in Obesity Research 1990*. John Libbey, London, pp. 659–661.

Berger M, Berchtold P (1978). The so-called ideal body weight. *Dtsch Med Wschr* 103: 1495.

Berger M, Müller W A, Renold A E (1978). Relationship of obesity to diabetes: some facts, many questions. In: Katzen H M, Mahler R J (eds) *Advances in Modern Nutrition*, Vol. III. Hemisphere, Washington DC, pp. 211–228.

Berger M, Berchtold P, Gries F A, Zimmermann H (1980). Indications for the treatment of obesity. In: Björntorp P, Cairella M, Howard A N (eds) *Recent Advances in Obesity Research*, Vol. III. John Libbey, London, pp. 1–9.

Berger M, Jörgens V, Kemmer F W, Berchtold P (1983). Health hazards of obesity. In: Kevany J (ed.) *Energy Balance in Human Nutrition*. Royal Irish Academy, Dublin, pp. 58–64.

Garrow J S, Wooley S C, Garner D M (1994). Should obesity be treated? *British Medical Journal* **309**: 654.

Gortmaker S L, Must A, Perrrin J M *et al.* (1993). Social and economic consequences of overweight in adolescence and young adulthood. *New England Journal of Medicine* **329**: 1208.

Gries F A, Berchtold P, Berger M (1976*). Adipositas. Pathophysiologie, Klinik, Therapie.* Springer, Berlin.

Isles C G (1992). The Renfrew and Paisley survey. *Lancet* **339**: 702.

Klesse R, Berchtold, P, Berger M (1980). Mortality of obese patients: the Düsseldorf mortality study (abstract). *Alimentazione Nutr Metabolismo* **1**: 291.

Kuczmarski R J, Flegal K M, Campbell S M, Johnson C L (1994). Increasing prevalence of overweight among US adults. *Journal of the American Medical Association* **272**: 205.

Lee, I-M, Manson J E, Hennekens C H, Paffenbarger R S (1993). Body weight and mortality. *Journal of the American Medical Association* **270**: 2823.

Lissner L, Odell P M, D'Agostino R B *et al.* (1991). Variability of body weight and health outcomes in the Framingham population. *New England Journal of Medicine* **324**: 1839.

Metropolitan Life Insurance Company (1959). New weight standards for men and women. *Stat Bull Metropol Life Ins Co* **40**: 1.

O'Sullivan J B (1982). Body weight and subsequent diabetes mellitus. *Journal of the American Medical Association* **248**: 949.

Rissanen A, Heliövaara M, Knekt P *et al.* (1989). Weight and mortality in Finnish men. *Journal of Clinical Epidemiology* **42**: 781.

Society of Actuaries (1959, 1960). *Build and Blood Pressure Study*, Part I, 1959; Part II 1960. Society of Actuaries, Chicago.

Society of Actuaries (1980). *The Build Study 1979*. Society of Actuaries, Chicago.

Trautner C, Haastert B, Berger M *et al.* (1994). Predictors of mortality in a large cohort of obese patients: multivariate analysis (abstract). *International Journal of Obesity* **18** (Suppl. 2): 54.

West K M (1978). *Epidemiology of Diabetes and its Vascular Lesions.* Elsevier/North Holland, New York.

White A, Nicholas G, Foster G. Browne F, Carey S (1993). *Health Survey for England 1991*. Office of Population Censuses and Surveys. London.

CHAPTER 2

Are all calories equal?

Andrew M. Prentice

INTRODUCTION

This chapter will address the deceptively simple question 'Are all calories equal?' and will examine whether the source of energy in the diet has any influence on weight control, on the development of obesity or on slimming. It will attempt to determine whether, in these days of abundant food supplies in affluent societies, it makes any difference what proportion of dietary energy comes from each of the major energy-yielding macronutrients: fat, carbohydrate, protein and alcohol. This question is central to the development, either at the public health or at the individual level, of strategies to prevent the encroaching epidemic of obesity.

A number of epidemiological studies provide evidence that all calories are not equal, and that a high fat–carbohydrate ratio in the diet plays a key role in undermining body weight regulatory systems in man (Dreon *et al.*, 1988; Romieu *et al.*, 1988; Tremblay *et al.*, 1989; Miller *et al.*, 1990; Gazzaniga and Burns, 1991; Tucker and Kano, 1992; Bolton-Smith and Woodward, 1994; Hill and Prentice, 1995). If this is the case, the key question is where, in the regulation of metabolism and energy intake, the macronutrients might exert different effects on energy balance.

Over the past 50 years there has been a rise of about 3 BMI units in the weight of the British population, indicating that the average adult is now over 10 kg heavier at an equivalent height, and the proportion of people who are classified as clinically obese has doubled in the last 10 years (Knight, 1984; White *et al.*, 1993). Similar changes have occurred in the United States (Kuczmarski *et al.*, 1994). Since the gene pool has remained essentially constant in this short period, it is evident that environmental and behavioural changes must represent the largest contributors to this problem. The transition to a

Weight Control
Edited by Richard Cottrell.
Published in 1995 by Chapman & Hall, London. ISBN 0 412 73600 4

generally sedentary lifestyle seems a likely contributor, but dietary changes, which are particularly well documented in the UK, also seem very likely to be implicated. Longitudinal studies demonstrate that since the Second World War there has been a rise in the proportion of dietary energy derived from fat (from 32% to a peak of 42%, Figure 2.1), and a reciprocal decrease in carbohydrate, changes that parallel the increase in BMI (Ministry of Agriculture, Fisheries and Food, 1994).

Evidence that these similar secular trends might be causally linked comes from cross-sectional analyses indicating that the selection of a diet with a high fat–carbohydrate ratio is associated with obesity (Dreon *et al.*, 1988; Romieu *et al.*, 1988; Tremblay *et al.*, 1989; Miller *et al.*, 1990; Gazzaniga and Burns, 1991; Tucker and Kano, 1992; Bolton-Smith and Woodward, 1994; Hill and Prentice, 1995).

Figure 2.2 shows an analysis by Bolton-Smith and Woodward (1994) of dietary data from over 11 600 Scottish men and women. These authors divided the sample into quintiles according to their intake of sugars and fat and the fat–sugar ratio, and examined the prevalence of obesity in each subgroup. Contrary to many people's prejudice, the groups consuming the most sugar had the lowest levels of obesity. This is almost certainly because of the so-called 'fat–sugar see-saw', i.e. people consuming most sugar (as a percentage of total energy) tend to consume the lowest ratio of fat and vice versa (Gibney and Lee, 1989). Thus, if we examine the data categorized by fat intake, and particularly by the fat–sugar ratio, it is apparent that the high fat consumers have a higher prevalence of obesity.

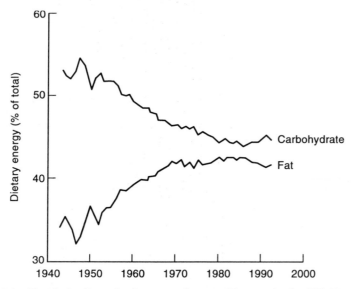

Figure 2.1 Trends in diet selection over the past 50 years in the UK. Data from National Food Surveys (Ministry of Agriculture, Fisheries and Food, 1994).

Are all calories equal?

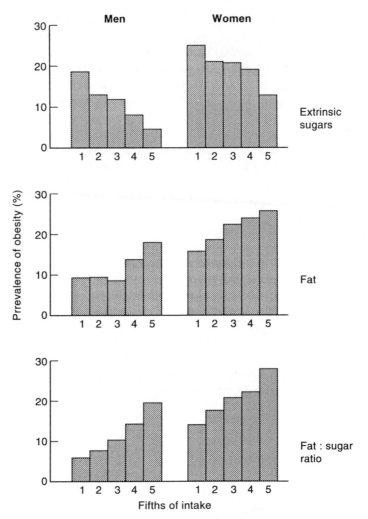

Figure 2.2 The impact of diet selection on the likelihood of developing obesity. Data from 11 626 men and women from the Scottish Heart Health and Scottish arm of MONICA studies. Quintile 1 = lowest intake. Redrawn from Bolton-Smith and Woodward (1993).

These and other data are very striking in implicating a high fat intake in the causation of obesity, but not everybody on a high-fat diet becomes obese. Evidently some are more susceptible than others, and there may be a number of reasons for this individual susceptibility.

In addition to dietary fat there has been a particular debate over the role of alcohol in the aetiology of obesity, with a number of conflicting data. Colditz *et al.* (1991) analysed the BMI of 85 000 nurses in America according to their daily alcohol intake. The analysis shows that BMI was greatest in the non-drinkers and declined with increasing alcohol consumption (Figure 2.3).

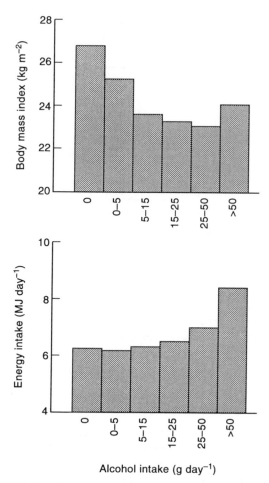

Figure 2.3 Relationship between alcohol intake and BMI in American women. Redrawn from Colditz *et al.* (1991).

Recorded energy intakes rise as alcohol intake rises, which suggests that alcohol is supplementing food intake and apparently not substituting for other foods. This paradoxical association between alcohol intake and fatness has been interpreted by some to indicate that alcohol calories are used very inefficiently by the organism (Lands and Zakhari, 1991; Leiber, 1991), thus supplying another example of how all calories might not be equal.

POSSIBLE MECHANISMS BY WHICH CALORIES FROM MACRONUTRIENTS MIGHT NOT BE EQUAL

There are a number of points in the physiological pathways leading from energy intake to ultimate storage at which macronutrients may differ (Figure 2.4). They may have different effects on hunger and satiety and thus

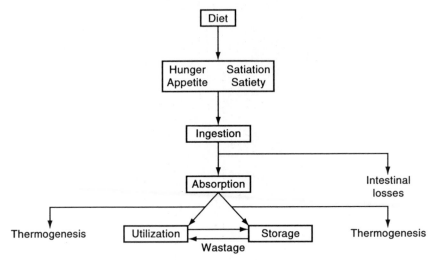

Figure 2.4 Points at which macronutrients may exert different effects on energy balance.

on the regulation of energy intake; they may be absorbed from the gut more or less efficiently; they might invoke different levels of diet-induced thermogenesis; or they may be utilized and stored with different levels of metabolic efficiency. These different possibilities are examined below.

Absorption of macronutrients

The classic Atwater data, updated by Southgate and Durnin (1970) demonstrate that energy is extracted very efficiently from food in healthy people (Table 2.1).

Available carbohydrates are completely absorbed while the amount of unabsorbed energy from dietary fibre or non-starch polysaccharides is low and variable. Around 9% of protein remains unabsorbed, with further losses in the urine due to its incomplete oxidation. Around 4% of fat and 2% of alcohol escapes absorption. With the exception of unavailable carbohydrates, these figures are low, and relatively similar for the different macronutrients. Furthermore the inter-individual differences are small.

Table 2.1 Digestible energy for the different macronutrients (expressed as a percentage of gross energy) (Carpenter, 1940; Southgate and Durnin, 1970)

Available carbohydrate	1.00
Unavailable carbohydrate	Variable
Protein	0.91
Fat	0.96
Alcohol	0.98

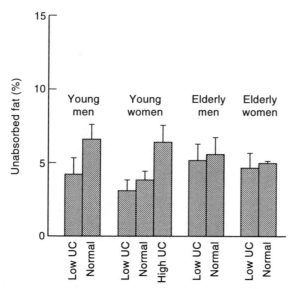

Figure 2.5   Efficiency of absorption of dietary fat. Error bars = SE. UC, unavailable carbohydrate. Data from Southgate and Durnin (1970).

Figure 2.5 shows data from the Southgate and Durnin studies in which unabsorbed fat was measured in groups of 12–16 young and elderly men and women who were fed diets with differing amounts of unavailable carbohydrate (Southgate and Durnin, 1970). The figure illustrates the very low levels of unabsorbed fat and the low level of variability indicated by the small standard errors. The standard errors are reduced even further when the data are expressed in terms of overall energy absorption. Thus, we can conclude that all macronutrients are very efficiently absorbed and that there is little variability between subjects that might help in explaining their differing susceptibility to obesity.

Macronutrient-induced thermogenesis

Studies of diet-induced thermogenesis generally show that, in the immediate post-meal period, less energy is dissipated as heat from the digestion of fat than from carbohydrate or protein (see, for example, Figure 2.6). This highlights a danger about fat calories: they are used with little dissipation of their energy.

The issue of thermogenesis is of particular relevance for alcohol since, if it is argued that alcohol calories do not count, they must be burnt off as heat, which should be readily measurable as a diet-induced thermogenesis approaching 100%. Figure 2.7 demonstrates that this is certainly not the case. In the immediate post-meal period very little energy is wasted as heat. Even when measured over the whole day the maximum recorded

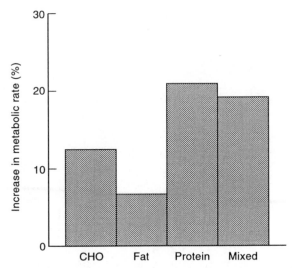

Figure 2.6 Diet-induced thermogenesis in response to ingestion of equicaloric loads of different macronutrients. Data from Swaminathan *et al.* (1985).

wastage of energy was 25% in the study of Suter *et al.* (1992), which provided over 14 units of alcohol per day. Our own study using slightly more realistic intakes of alcohol recorded only 14% wastage, which suggests that alcohol calories are used with a similar efficiency to carbohydrate calories (Sonko *et al.*, 1994).

A smaller number of studies have examined the effect of macronutrient manipulations on total 24-hour energy expenditure measured in a whole-body calorimeter.

Figure 2.8 shows data from a recent study in which the carbohydrate content of the diet was varied from 9% to 79% with reciprocal changes in fat intake (Shetty *et al.*, 1995). Despite this variation, in which macronutrient intake was manipulated at close to the limits of possibility using normal foodstuffs, this had no significant effect on daily energy expenditure or net energy balance. Thomas *et al.* (1992) have also demonstrated trivial differences in diet-induced thermogenesis when nutrient intake is manipulated within the normal limits of human diets. Figure 2.9 shows that in lean and obese men and women, although fuel selection differed, as indicated by the different respiratory quotients, energy expenditure was the same on high-, medium- or low-carbohydrate diets.

Interconversion of macronutrients

Classical biochemistry teaches that the macronutrients are inter-related in terms of their functional and storage sites, and, through oxidation via the tricarboxylic acid (TCA) cycle, they compete with each other in an oxidative hierarchy. In relation to obesity, one of the key questions is the extent

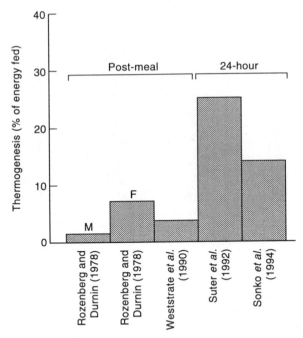

Figure 2.7 Diet-induced thermogenesis in response to alcohol ingestion. M, males; F, females. Data from Rozenberg and Durnin. (1978), Weststrate *et al.* (1990), Suter *et al.* (1992), Sonko *et al.* (1994).

to which fat is synthesized from carbohydrate. The necessary biochemical pathways certainly exist and are extensively utilized in animals such as rats

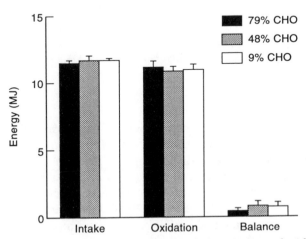

Figure 2.8 Similarity of 24-hour energy expenditure on diets of widely differing fat–carbohydrate ratios when fed to energy balance. Data from whole-body calorimetry (Shetty *et al.*, 1995). CHO, carbohydrate

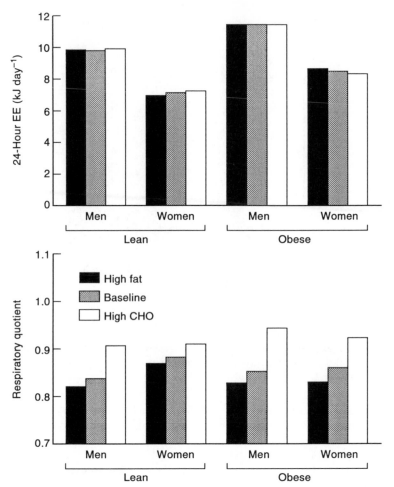

Figure 2.9 Similarity of 24-hour energy expenditure on diets of widely differing fat–carbohydrate ratios when fed *ad libitum*. Data from whole-body calorimetry (Thomas *et al.*, 1992).

fed on a low-fat 'chow' diet. Their relevance in humans who are already consuming large amounts of preformed fats is less clear.

The recent work by Hellerstein's group in California suggests that under normal circumstances (i.e. in lean people in energy balance) there is minimal fat synthesis in either the fasting or the post-prandial state (Figure 2.10) (Hellerstein *et al.*, 1991; Schwartz, 1993). Levels are somewhat higher in the hyperinsulinaemic obese after a meal but are still very low. When substantially overfed, people have little option but to convert some of the excess carbohydrate to fat and to store it, as indicated on the right-hand side of Figure 2.10.

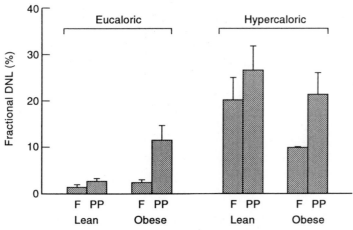

Figure 2.10 Extent of *de novo* lipogenesis (DNL) from carbohydrate in humans. Measurements made by [^{13}C]acetate tracer technique from J. M. Schwartz (personal communication). F, fasting; PP, postprandial.

These important data on low levels of fat synthesis offer further insights into why high-carbohydrate diets seem to be much less fattening than high-fat diets since energy is not such a readily interconvertible currency within the body as was formerly believed. In practice, human metabolism is very reluctant to turn carbohydrate into fat.

Macronutrient storage

Table 2.2 lists the estimated efficiency of storage of the various dietary fuels as fat (Blaxter, 1989). The efficiency with which dietary fat is deposited in adipose tissue is extraordinarily high, wasting only 4% of the energy, whereas fat storage from carbohydrate and protein dissipates 20% and 34% respectively. This is yet another reason why fat may be peculiarly adipogenic.

Net macronutrient balance

Finally, consideration must be given to the regulation of macronutrient balance. For a long time it was thought that, once nutrients had crossed

Table 2.2 Efficiency of macronutrient storage

Dietary substrate	Product	Estimated efficiency	Heat increment
Carbohydrate	Body fat	0.80	0.20
Protein	Body fat	0.66	0.34
Fat	Body fat	0.96	0.04
Carbohydrate	Glycogen	0.95	0.05
Protein	Body protein	0.86	0.14

Adapted from Blaxter (1989).

the intestinal lumen, all sources of energy formed a mutually interchange-
able energy currency and that the initial macronutrient source was of little
consequence. However, we now take a rather more sophisticated view in
which we believe that it is important to consider how the body balances
each of the macronutrients separately, within a hierarchy of metabolic
reactivity (Figure 2.11).

Alcohol comes at the top of the hierarchy because there is no ability to
store alcohol, and because it is essentially a toxin that must be oxidized
before it can be cleared from the body. Since total energy expenditure is
constant (except for the small amount of thermogenesis indicated in Figure
2.7), the oxidation of all other substrates must be suppressed when alcohol
is being burnt. This can be readily demonstrated in practice (Shelmet *et al.*,
1988; Sonko *et al.*, 1994). Carbohydrate and protein come next since they
have limited storage space in the body. There is a close linkage between
intake and oxidation. When extra carbohydrate is consumed its oxidation
increases in a very sensitive 'autoregulatory' manner in order to re-estab-
lish balance (Schutz *et al.*, 1989), and similarly for protein.

However, fat behaves quite differently. When extra fat is ingested, fat
oxidation hardly changes at all (Schutz *et al.*, 1989). Indeed, fat oxidation
is usually suppressed in response to an excess food intake and fat is stored
because the body oxidizes the excesses of the other macronutrients above
it in this hierarchy and fat oxidation takes the lowest priority.

An example of the excellent autoregulatory control of carbohydrate oxidation is shown in Figure 2.12. This shows data from a study performed
in whole-body calorimeters in which the fat–carbohydrate ratio of men's
diets was covertly manipulated, leaving the protein level constant (Shetty
et al., 1995). This provides evidence of a very sensitive autoregulatory
adjustment of carbohydrate oxidation to match intake levels and maintain
a rather constant balance in the face of even extreme dietary manipulations.
Fat oxidation also appears to be responding in an accurate autoregulatory
way, but this is simply because fat oxidation alters in a reciprocal manner
to carbohydrate in order to make up the remaining metabolic energy need.
This claim is supported by data from a multitude of experiments.

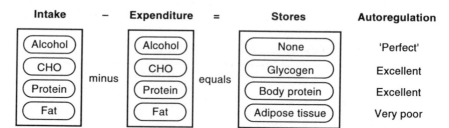

Figure 2.11 Scheme describing macronutrient balance equations in terms of the
oxidative hierarchy. Note that there is no particular significance to the order in
which carbohydrate and protein are illustrated; both show good autoregulation.
The key feature is that fat is at the bottom of the hierarchy.

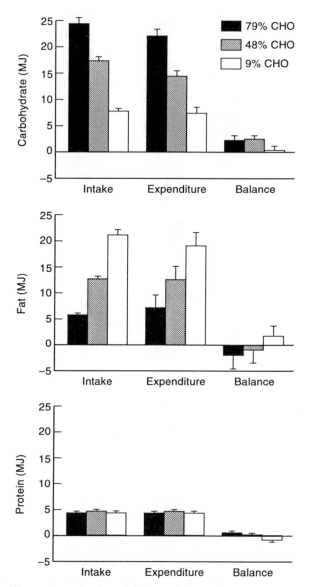

Figure 2.12 Illustration of autoregulatory adjustments in carbohydrate oxidation in response to changes in intake. See text for interpretation. Data from whole-body calorimeter measurements (Shetty *et al.*, 1995).

For example, Figure 2.13 shows an experiment in which volunteers were overfed and underfed carbohydrate for 7 days while fat was held constant, and overfed and underfed fat while carbohydrate was held constant (McNeill *et al.*, 1992). When carbohydrate intake was manipulated the carbohydrate oxidation rate responded to almost the same extent, while fat oxidation was forced in the opposite direction. In contrast, when the

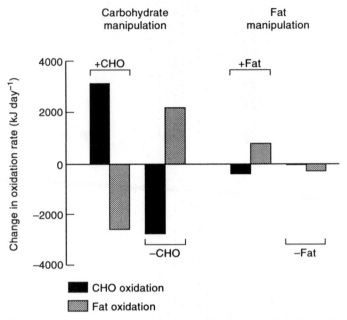

Figure 2.13 Experiments indicating that carbohydrate, rather than fat, drives adjustments in fuel selection. See text for description of methods and interpretation. Horizontal lines indicate extent of manipulations. Data from McNeill *et al.* (1992).

manipulations were achieved by adding and subtracting energy as fat there is virtually no response. Once again it seems as if the system is effectively blind to differences in fat intake. Carbohydrate is well regulated, yet fat is poorly regulated.

In summary, because of the body's virtually unlimited capacity to store fat there is no automatic compensatory system that attempts to match oxidation rates to intake in the manner that exists for the other macronutrients. Furthermore, the macronutrient hierarchy indicates that fat balance is poorly regulated because it is always dominated by the body's greater need to regulate its very limited glycogen stores (Flatt, 1987).

Thus it appears that post-ingestive differences in macronutrients are small; differences in absorption efficiency between fuels and between individuals are quite minor, 24-hour energy expenditure is remarkably unaffected by profound changes in diet composition and the body is very effective at adjusting the mix of fuels that it oxidizes (the respiratory quotient, RQ) to match the mixture ingested (the food quotient, FQ).

This implies that if people eat to energy balance the choice of diet will have little effect on body weight. This in turn implies that the major effects seen in cross-sectional surveys, indicating that high-fat diets are implicated in the development of obesity, must be mediated through the dysregulation of food intake.

Macronutrient effects on appetite

Most research on this topic has been conducted using a variation of the classic preload design in which subjects are given an initial meal that can be covertly loaded with different macronutrients. Subjects are then asked to complete visual analogue ratings for hunger and satiety, and after a fixed interval are invited to eat freely from a second 'outcome' meal. In many of these experiments food intake for the remainder of the day is self-recorded by the volunteers in a diary. The consensus of information from the literature in this field is that protein is most satiating and fat is least satiating. Indeed, fat is often claimed to have virtually no satiating power at all. However, there is by no means a total consensus.

Figure 2.14 shows data from a study generally accepted as supporting the view that fat fails to elicit a compensatory decrease in subsequent intake (Caputo and Mattes, 1992). The authors conclude that when the excess preload is given as carbohydrate, intake is suppressed over the rest of the day so that there is no significant difference in overall energy intake between the low and high preloads or the control treatment. On the other hand, when the excess is provided as fat the total intake over the day was significantly elevated because of a failure to compensate. However, close examination of the figure reveals that this claim is based on two rather similar effects differing only in the fact that the effect was significant for fat and not for carbohydrate. In contrast, in a study by de-Graaf *et al.* (Figure 2.15)

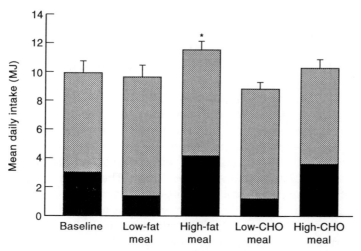

Figure 2.14 Adjustments in voluntary food intake in response to covert preloads of differing energy and macronutrient content (fat less satiating). Solid bars represent intake from preload, hatched bars represent intake over remainder of the day. Reproduced from Caputo and Mattes (1992) Human dietary responses to covert manipulation of energy, fat and carbohydrate in a midday meal, *American Journal of Clinical Nutrition*, **56**: 36–43, © *American Journal of Clinical Nutrition*, American Society for Clinical Nutrition, with permission.

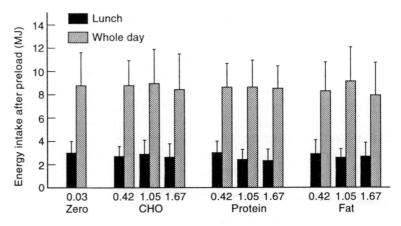

Figure 2.15 Adjustments in voluntary food intake in response to covert preloads of differing energy and macronutrient content (no effect of different macronutrients). Reproduced from de-Graaf *et al.* (1992) Short-term effects of different amounts of protein, fats and carbohydrates on satiety, *American Journal of Clinical Nutrition*, **55**: 33–38, © *American Journal of Clinical Nutrition*, American Society for Clinical Nutrition, with permission.

none of the preloads, given as carbohydrate, protein or fat, and at different levels of intake, had any significant effect on energy intake at the following lunch or over the remainder of the day (de-Graaf *et al.*, 1992).

Some of these differences may be related to variations in the study design, including the size of the preload, the time elapsed before the test meal and the diet selection available at this time.

Figure 2.16 shows clearly that the satiating effects of the various macronutrients vary according to the size of the preload (Weststrate, 1992). At a preload of 250 kcal fat actually appears to be the most satiating and protein the least, although the differences may not be significant. At 400 kcal the generally accepted order of satiety emerges with protein above carbohydrate and fat at the bottom. Note that it requires a preload of around 800 kcal of fat to be as satiating as 400 kcal carbohydrate, and that 800 kcal fat is much less satiating than 400 kcal protein. The discrepancies between various studies might also be partly resolved by recent observations that certain subgroups of people (e.g. restrained eaters and the obese) are especially insensitive to the satiating effects of fat (Rolls *et al.*, 1994). This would obscure the relationships within any groups that had not been carefully characterized with respect to such variables.

Our own studies have taken the view that in order to sort out the controversy it is preferable to conduct studies over a longer period, and to be able to measure the true effects on fat balance. These studies have been performed within the confines of a whole-body calorimeter which in some respects provides an ideal setting, offering quiet and reproducible conditions, with

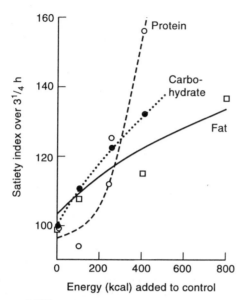

Figure 2.16 Effects of different macronutrients on satiety index, calculated as area under visual analogue ratings curves compared with control treatment. Data from Weststrate (1992).

a minimum of external eating cues, making it possible to be absolutely certain what the subject has eaten. Our calorimeters allow changes in macronutrient balance to be monitored to ±20 g day^{-1} for carbohydrate and ±10 g day^{-1} for fat (Murgatroyd *et al.*, 1993).

In the first experiment six lean men each spent three periods of 7 days in the whole-body calorimeters (Stubbs *et al.*, 1993a, 1995a).They had *ad libitum* access to food in both timing and quantity, but not to food type, which was covertly manipulated to provide 20%, 40% or 60% energy from fat. These diets were offered in random order.

Figure 2.17 shows the effect of these covert manipulations on fat balance in one of the subjects. Fat balance is calculated relative to a nominal zero at the beginning of each week by continuously cumulating fat intake at each meal (shown by the ascending lines) and fat oxidation (shown by the descending line), which is calculated from the respiratory gas exchanges. On the 20% fat diet this subject was in negative fat balance. On the 40% diet his fat balance was slightly positive and on the 60% diet he gained 700 g of pure fat in just 7 days. The mean results for the whole group showed a similar pattern. On the low-fat diet there was a spontaneous loss of body fat, while on the 60% fat diet there was massive fat gain. It appears that the subjects' appetite control systems did not recognize that they were ingesting excess energy on the high-fat diet, so that instead of reducing their food intake they continued to eat a very similar weight of food on each of the three experimental diets and consequently consumed much

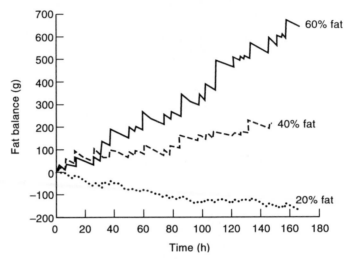

Figure 2.17 Effect of covert manipulations of fat–carbohydrate ratio of diets on fat balance. Fat balance calculated as the cumulative sum of fat intake from meals (ascending lines) and fat oxidation (descending lines) calculated from respiratory gas exchange measured in a whole-body calorimeter over three different 7-day periods. Data from Stubbs *et al.* (1995).

more fat on the 60% fat diet than on the 20%. This is a dramatic illustration of the phenomenon of 'passive overconsumption' since subjects were not actually eating a greater volume of food.

It may be argued that these results were influenced by the artificial nature of the calorimeter environment, but similar results have been obtained under free-living conditions, measured over 14 days per diet. Fat balance was not measured directly since data were not available on the respiratory quotients, but energy balance was measured by simultaneous measures of energy expenditure using the doubly labelled water method (Stubbs *et al.*, 1993b,1995b).

Figure 2.18 shows that the 'treatment' effect (indicated by the trend across treatments) was exactly the same as we had previously noted, but overall energy balance was less positive, presumably because the subjects were more active outside the calorimeter. As previously, the subjects continued to consume very similar amounts of food on each diet because their physiology failed to detect the excess. Even after 14 days there appeared to be almost no tendency for the intakes to adapt on the different diets, suggesting a lack of any 'physiological learning' process.

These experiments provide clear evidence for high-fat hyperphagia, the so-called passive overconsumption or, expressed another way, a failure of down-regulation of food intake in response to a high-fat diet. The key question is whether it is the fat *per se* that is causing the overeating or simply the fact that high-fat diets tend to be much more energy dense than low-fat diets.

To test this we performed a third experiment in which the fat content of the

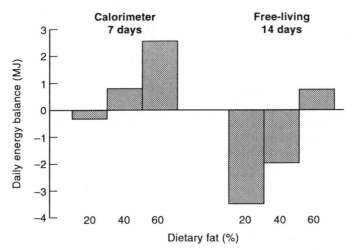

Figure 2.18 Effect of covert manipulations of fat–carbohydrate ratio of diets on energy balance measured under confined and free-living conditions. Data from six subjects (Stubbs *et al.*,1995a, b).

foods was manipulated as before but in addition the energy density of the diets was held constant (Stubbs and Prentice, 1993).

Figure 2.19 demonstrates that in this situation the high-fat hyperphagia detected in the two previous studies was abolished. This suggests that the energy density of foods may be a more critical determinant of energy intake than the fat content. In practical terms for individuals consuming 'off-the-shelf' foods, this distinction may be academic since energy density and fat content of foods are so highly correlated. However, it may provide an

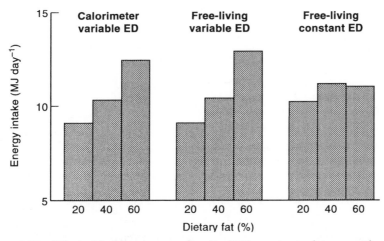

Figure 2.19 Effect of holding energy density (ED) constant when covertly manipulating the fat–carbohydrate ratio of diets. Data from six subjects (Stubbs and Prentice, 1993; Stubbs *et al.*, 1995a, b).

important clue to the metabolic details of the regulatory processes.

The role of macronutrients in the regulation of appetite is clearly complex. Although there is a general consensus that satiety effects are greatest for protein and least for fat, the literature is by no means conclusive in this area. (Incidentally, the position of alcohol in this respect is particularly unclear.) It is also often stated that 'up-regulation' is more efficient than 'down-regulation', suggesting that we may be better at protecting ourselves against hunger than we are against an excess of food. This would make good teleological sense in terms of survival. Finally high-fat (high-energy foods) lead to passive overconsumption because satiety signals fail to compensate.

But what are the practical consequences of these observations for slimmers? Is there a metabolic rationale for the prescription of a low-fat diet to achieve weight loss?

ARE ALL CALORIES EQUAL FOR SLIMMERS?

The inverse rationale to the theory of passive overconsumption would simply be that if we can persuade people to consume a diet with a reduced fat content and hence reduced energy density, and if their regulatory systems fail to recognize this and to adjust food intake, then they will lose weight.

Figure 2.20 shows data from a number of studies in which the energy density of foods was covertly altered and the ability of individuals to compensate was tested. The solid circles show the degree of energy manipulation and the open circles the subsequent intake. If people were good at detecting the manipulation, and if compensation had been perfect, the resultant intake would be 100%. However, the fact that the open circles lie close to the closed

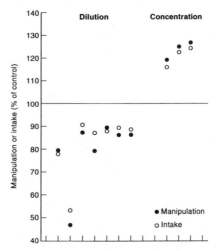

Figure 2.20 Experiments testing the efficiency of dietary compensation in response to manipulation of the energy content of foods. Data from Glueck *et al.* (1982), Duncan *et al.* (1987), Lissner *et al.* (1987), Tremblay *et al.* (1989), Kendall *et al.* (1991), Stubbs *et al.* (1993a, b; 1995a, b).

circles indicates a failure of compensation. This compilation of results refutes the suggestion made previously that 'up-regulation' is better than 'down-regulation', since there appears to be little difference. However, this is good news in terms of dieting since, for dieting to be successful, we do not want slimmers to compensate automatically for caloric dilution.

There are now a number of studies in the literature in which volunteers have consumed *ad libitum* diets.

Figure 2.21 shows data from Lissner *et al.* (1987), who investigated the effect

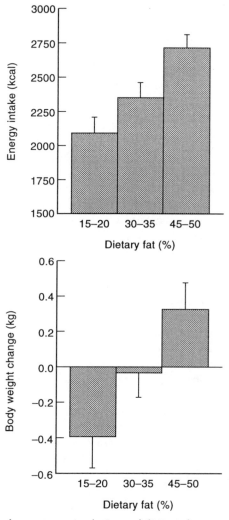

Figure 2.21 Effect of covert manipulations of dietary fat on spontaneous food intake (a) and changes in body weight (b) over 2 weeks. Reproduced from Lissner *et al.* (1987) Dietary fat and the regulation of energy intake in human subjects, *American Journal of Clinical Nutrition*, **46**: 886–892, © *American Journal of Clinical Nutrition*, American Society for Clinical Nutrition, with permission.

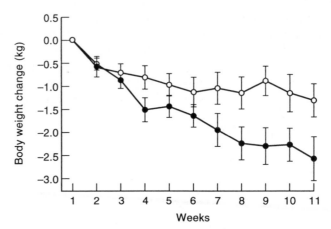

Figure 2.22 Effect of covert manipulations of dietary fat on spontaneous food intake and cumulative weight loss (mean ± SEM) over 11 weeks. ○, Control; ●, low-fat diet. Reproduced from Kendall *et al.* (1991) Weight loss on a low fat diet: consequences of the imprecision of the control of food intake in humans, *American Journal of Clinical Nutrition*, **53**: 1124–1129, © *American Journal of Clinical Nutrition*, American Society for Clinical Nutrition, with permission.

of covert manipulation of the diet. Energy intake was lower on a low-fat diet and weight loss occurred spontaneously. The actual effect on body fat may have been greater than suggested by the changes in body weight since the low-fat diet, which was high in carbohydrate, may have caused some glycogen loading and water retention, and vice versa for the high-fat diet, attenuating the weight change. A follow-up study by Kendall *et al.* (1991), conducted over 11 weeks, showed similar results (Figure 2.22), with a mean loss of 2.5 kg in the low-fat group compared with 1.1 kg in the control group.

Although the weight loss in these studies is not large in terms of the goals of most slimmers, these experiments were carried out in normal people who had no planned intention of losing weight.

Low-fat diets have also been used in weight maintenance programmes.

Figure 2.23 shows that the group trained to consume a low-fat diet was marginally better off than the control group, showing no weight regain by 12 months, but the difference was not very great (Toubro and Astrup, 1994). However, the key question is whether low-fat *ad libitum* diets are any more or less effective than a traditional calorie-counting regimen. Studies such as that of Schlundt *et al.* (1993) suggest that the answer may well be 'no'. Figure 2.24 shows that there was a similar loss of fat-free tissue, but a greater weight loss and hence fat loss, on a traditional calorie-restricted diet.

However, we should perhaps take a longer term view since the study of Shah *et al.* (1994) (Figure 2.25) shows that, although weight loss was very similar on low-fat and energy-restricted diets the low-fat diet was much more acceptable to the patients and therefore might be adhered to longer as a permanent modification to their eating habits.

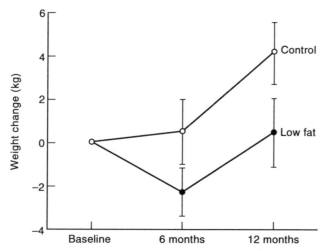

Figure 2.23 Effect of a low-fat diet on weight maintenance after treatment with a very low-energy diet. Data from Toubro and Astrup (1994).

To summarize, with respect to low-fat diets and weight control, it seems that the balance of evidence is that low-fat diets do aid weight loss and such diets are likely to have other health benefits. Perhaps the chief limitation to their effectiveness is our inability to persuade people to modify their diets.

'ARE ALL CALORIES EQUAL?'

The evidence suggests that in terms of absorption and metabolism humans cope efficiently over a wide range of diets. Thus, in this respect, calories

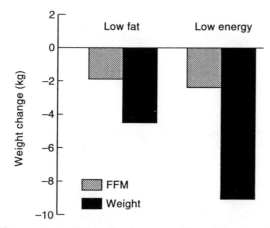

Figure 2.24 Comparison of the effectiveness of low-fat and traditional calorie-counting low-energy diets. Data from Schlundt *et al.* (1993). FFM, fat-free mass.

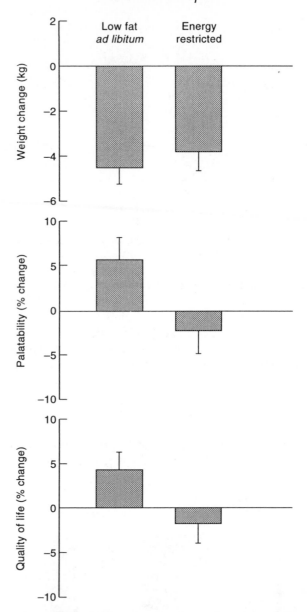

Figure 2.25 Effects of an *ad libitum* low-fat diet and traditional low-energy diet on palatability and quality of life. Data from Shah *et al.* (1994).

may be considered relatively equal so long as they are consumed to energy balance. The main differences between macronutrients are probably mediated through the regulation of food intake; certainly high-fat diets easily cause passive overconsumption of energy, but this may, in fact, be a consequence of the energy density of foods as much as their macronutrient composition. There is considerable experimental evidence that high-fat, high-energy diets undermine the weight regulatory systems of humans and promote obesity. In contrast, high-carbohydrate diets seem relatively benign, and in this respect they seem to have a useful role to play in the long-term prevention and treatment of obesity.

REFERENCES

Blaxter K (1989). *Energy Metabolism in Animals and Man*. Cambridge University Press, Cambridge.

Bolton-Smith C, Woodward M (1993). The prevalence of overweight and obesity in different fat and sugar consumption groups. *Proceedings of the Nutrition Society* **52**: 383A.

Bolton-Smith C, Woodward M (1994). Dietary composition and fat to sugar ratios in relation to obesity. *International Journal of Obesity* **18**: 820–828.

Caputo F A, Mattes R D (1992). Human dietary responses to covert manipulations of energy, fat and carbohydrate in a midday meal. *American Journal of Clinical Nutrition* **56**: 36–43.

Carpenter T M (1940). The metabolism of alcohol: a review. *Quarterly Journal of Studies on Alcohol* **1**: 201–226.

Colditz G A, Giovannucci E, Rimm E B *et al*. (1991). Alcohol intake in relation to diet and obesity in women and men. *American Journal of Clinical Nutrition* **54**: 49–55.

de-Graaf C, Hulshof T, Westrate J A, Jas P (1992). Short-term effects of different amounts of protein, fats and carbohydrates on satiety. *American Journal of Clinical Nutrition* **55**: 33–38.

Dreon D M, Frey-Hewitt B, Ellsworth N *et al*. (1988). Dietary fat:carbohydrate ratio and obesity in middle-aged men. *American Journal of Clinical Nutrition* **47**: 995–1000.

Duncan K H, Bacon J A, Weinsier R L (1987). The effects of high and low energy density diets on satiety, energy intake and eating time of obese and non-obese subjects. *American Journal of Clinical Nutrition* **46**: 886–892.

Flatt J P (1987). The difference in the storage capacities for carbohydrate and for fat, and its implications in the regulation of body weight. *Annals of the New York Academy of Sciences* **499**: 104–123.

Gazzaniga J M, Burns T L (1991). The relationship between diet composition and body fatness in pre-adolescent children. *Journal of the American Dietetic Association* **91** (Supplement): A-63.

Gibney M J, Lee P (1989). Patterns of food and nutrient intake in adults consuming high and low levels of table sugar in a Dublin suburb of chronically high unemployment. *Proceedings of the Nutrition Society* **48**: 132A.

Glueck C J, Hastings M M, Allen C *et al*. (1982). Sucrose polyester and covert caloric dilution. *American Journal of Clinical Nutrition* **35**: 1352–1359.

Hellerstein M K, Christiansen M, Kaempler S *et al*. (1991). Measurement of *de novo* hepatic lipogenesis in humans using stable isotopes. *Journal of Clinical Investigation* **87**: 1841–1852.

Hill J O, Prentice A M (1995). Sugars and body weight. *American Journal of Clinical Nutrition* **62** (Supplement), 178S–194S.

Kendall A, Levitsky D A, Strupp B J, Lissner L (1991). Weight loss on a low-fat diet: consequence of the imprecision of the control of food intake in humans. *American Journal of Clinical Nutrition* **53**: 1124–1129.

Knight I (1984). *The Heights and Weights of Adults in Great Britain*. OPCS/HMSO, London.

Kuczmarski R J, Flegal K M, Campbell S M, Johnson C L (1994). Increasing prevalence of overweight among US adults: The National Health and Nutrition Examination Surveys 1960 to 1991. *Journal of the American Medical Association* **272**: 205–211.

Lands W E M, Zakhari S (1987). The case of the missing calories. *American Journal of Clinical Nutrition* **54**: 47–48.

Leiber C S (1991). Perspectives: do alcohol calories count? *American Journal of Clinical Nutrition* **54**: 976–982.

Lissner L, Levitsky D A, Strupp, B J et al. (1987) Dietary fat and the regulation of energy intake in human subjects. *American Journal of Clinical Nutrition* **46**: 886–892.

McNeill G, Morrison D C, Davidson L, Smith J S (1992). The effect of changes in dietary carbohydrate v fat intake on 24-h energy expenditure and nutrient oxidation in post-menopausal women. *Proceedings of the Nutrition Society* **51**: 91A.

Miller W C, Linderman A K, Wallace J, Niederprum M (1990). Diet composition, energy intake and exercise in relation to body fat in men and women. *American Journal of Clinical Nutrition* **52**: 426–430.

Ministry of Agriculture, Fisheries and Food (1994). *Household Food Consumption and Expenditure*. HMSO, London, pp. 1940–1994.

Murgatroyd P R, Sonko B J, Wittekind A et al. (1993). Non-invasive techniques for assessing carbohydrate flux. 1. Measurement of depletion by indirect calorimetry. *Acta Physiologica Scandinavica* **147**: 91–98.

Rolls B J, Kim-Harris S, Fischman M W et al. (1994). Satiety after preloads with different amounts of fat and carbohydrate: implications for obesity. *American Journal of Clinical Nutrition* **60**: 476–487.

Romieu I, Willett W C, Stampfer M J et al. (1988). Energy intake and other determinants of relative weight. *American Journal of Clinical Nutrition* **47**: 406–412.

Rozenberg K, Durnin J V G A (1978). The effect of alcohol on resting metabolic rate. *British Journal of Nutrition* **40**: 293–298.

Schlundt D G, Hill J O, Pope-Cordle J et al. (1993). Randomized evaluation of a low fat ad libitum carbohydrate diet for weight reduction. *International Journal of Obesity* **17**: 623–629.

Schutz Y, Flatt J P, Jequier E (1989). Failure of dietary fat intake to promote fat oxidation: a factor favouring the development of obesity. *American Journal of Clinical Nutrition* **50**: 307–314.

Shah M, McGovern P, French S, Baxter J (1994). Comparison of a low-fat, ad libitum complex-carbohydrate diet with a low-energy diet in moderately obese women. *American Journal of Clinical Nutrition* **59**: 980–984.

Shelmet J J, Reichard G A, Skutches C L et al.(1988). Ethanol causes acute inhibition of carbohydrate, fat and protein oxidation and insulin resistance. *Journal of Clinical Investigation* **81**: 1137–1145.

Shetty P S, Prentice A M, Goldberg G R et al. (1994) Alterations in fuel selection and voluntary food intake in response to iso-energetic manipulation of glycogen stores in man. *American Journal of Clinical Nutrition* **60**, 534–543.

Sonko B J, Prentice A M, Murgatroyd P R et al. (1994). The influence of alcohol on postmeal fat storage. *American Journal of Clinical Nutrition* **59**: 619–625.

Southgate D A T, Durnin J V G A (1970). Calorie conversion factors: an experimental reassessment of the factors used in the calculation of the energy value of human diets. *British Journal of Nutrition* **24**: 517–535.

Stubbs R J, Prentice A M (1993). The effect of covertly manipulating the dietary fat:carbohydrate ratio of isoenergetically dense diets on ad lib intake in 'free-living' humans. *Proceedings of the Nutrition Society* **52**: 341A.

Stubbs R J, Murgatroyd P R, Goldberg G R, Prentice A M (1993a). The effect of covert manipulation of dietary fat and energy density on *ad libitum* food intake in humans. *Proceedings of the Nutrition Society* **52**: 35A.

Stubbs R J, Ritz P, Coward W A, Prentice A M (1993b). The effect of covert manipulation of dietary fat and energy density on ad libitum food intake in 'free-living' humans. *Proceedings of the Nutrition Society* **52**: 348A.

Stubbs R J, Harbron C G, Murgatroyd P R, Prentice A M (1995a). Covert manipulation of dietary fat and energy density: effect on substrate flux and food intake in men feeding *ad libitum*. *American Journal of Clinical Nutrition* **62**: 316–329.

Stubbs R J, Ritz P, Coward W A, Prentice A M (1995b). Covert manipulation of the dietary fat to carbohydrate ratio and energy density: effect on food intake and energy balance in free-living men, feeding ad libitum. *American Journal of Clinical Nutrition* **62**: 330–332.

Suter P M, Schutz Y, Jequier E (1992). The effect of ethanol on fat storage in healthy subjects. *New England Journal of Medicine* **326**: 983–987.

Swaminathan R, King R F G J, Holmfield J et al. (1985). Thermic effect of feeding carbohydrate, fat, protein, and mixed meal in lean and obese subjects. *American Journal of Clinical Nutrition* **42**: 177–181.

Thomas C D, Peters J C, Reed G W et al. (1992). Nutrient balance and energy expenditure during *ad libitum* feeding of high-fat and high-carbohydrate diets in humans. *American Journal of Clinical Nutrition* **55**: 934–942.

Toubro S, Astrup A (1994). Dietary weight maintenance: low-fat, high-carbohydrate *ad libitum* versus calorie counting (abstract). *International Journal of Obesity* **18** (Supplement 2): 123.

Tremblay A, Plourde G, Despres J-P, Bouchard C (1989). Impact of dietary fat content and fat oxidation on energy intake in humans. *American Journal of Clinical Nutrition* **49**: 799–805.

Tucker L A, Kano M J (1992). Dietary fat and body fat: a multivariate study of 205 adult females. *American Journal of Clinical Nutrition* **56**: 616–622.

Weststrate J A (1992). *Effect of Nutrients on the Regulation of Food Intake*. Unilever Research, Vlaardingen, The Netherlands.

Weststrate J A, Wunnink I, Duerenberg P, Hautvast J G A J (1990). Alcohol and its acute effects on resting metabolic rate and diet-induced thermogenesis. *British Journal of Nutrition* **64**: 413–425.

White A, Nicolaas G, Foster K et al. (1993). *Health Survey for England 1991*. OPCS/HMSO, London.

CHAPTER 3

Metabolic risk factors for the development of obesity

Arne Astrup, Anne Raben, Annebeth R. Skov, Claudia Sørensen and Søren Toubro

INTRODUCTION

The high, and increasing, prevalence of obesity in affluent societies has become a major health problem. Obesity commonly occurs as part of a metabolic syndrome that may show one or more manifestations, such as hyperlipidaemia, non-insulin-dependent (type II) diabetes mellitus, hypertension and atherosclerosis, either alone or in concert, causing ischaemic heart disease, stroke and premature mortality. Despite a wide range of efforts to prevent obesity, the prevalence of both moderate overweight and obesity is still increasing. An improved understanding of the mechanisms causing obesity seems necessary if efforts to prevent and treat overweight and obesity are to be successful. This review will deal with three genetically determined traits predisposing to weight gain: low relative resting energy expenditure expressed when sympathetic activity is suppressed by a low dietary carbohydrate content; low fat oxidation, which becomes significant when the fat content of the diet is high; and a taste preference for high-fat food items. In concert, these risk factors favour a positive fat balance and, over time, lead to obesity.

DETERMINANTS OF ENERGY EXPENDITURE

Most of the variation between individuals in energy expenditure (EE) is due to differences in body composition and level of physical activity. Up

Weight Control
Edited by Richard Cottrell.
Published in 1995 by Chapman & Hall, London. ISBN 0 412 73600 4

to 85% of the variation in resting EE (REE) can be accounted for by differences in fat-free mass (FFM) and fat mass (FM), whereas another 10% can be explained by differences in plasma concentrations of triiodothyronine and androstenedione, sympathetic nervous system (SNS) activity and body temperature (Ravussin and Bogardus, 1989). Age, gender, physical fitness and genetics account for some of the residual variation, and their impact on REE may be exerted through differences in sizes of organs and tissues making up the FFM.

Because the absolute REE is positively correlated with FFM, obesity is clearly associated with a high absolute REE. A low energy expenditure for a given body size and composition (relative EE) figures among the genetically determined factors that may contribute to weight gain (see later). In a cross-sectional study of Pima Indians, Bogardus *et al.* (1986) reported that 83% of the variance of REE could be accounted for by FFM, age and gender. Moreover, they reported that family membership accounted for an additional 11%, so that 94% of the total variability of REE could be explained. Together with support from twin studies, these results suggest that the relative REE is, at least partly, genetically determined (Bouchard *et al.*, 1989).

Since these studies were reported, other determinants of EE have been identified, such as sympathetic nervous system (SNS) activity (Saad *et al.*, 1991; Astrup *et al.*, 1992a; Spraul *et al.*, 1993), plasma concentrations of triiodothyronine (T_3) (Astrup *et al.*, 1992) and androstendione (Astrup *et al.*, 1992b; Svendsen *et al.*, 1993), body temperature (Rising *et al.*, 1992), physical training (Poehlman *et al.*, 1988) and muscle metabolism (Zurlo *et al.*, 1990a), and it is possible that variability in the genetic component of EE may be caused by differences in one or more of these determinants. In order to examine to what extent SNS activity and thyroid and androgen hormones could account for a possible familial component of EE, we have recently studied whether a familial component of 24-hour EE and REE could be found in 72 Caucasian siblings from 32 randomly selected families. We found that differences in FFM, FM, plasma noradrenaline, plasma T_3 and spontaneous physical activity were all significant determinants of 24-hour EE and could explain more than 90% of the variation in 24-hour EE between individuals. Twenty-four-hour EE adjusted for differences in FFM, FM, plasma noradrenaline, plasma T_3 and spontaneous physical activity, however, was not found to be a familial trait as no sibling pair resemblance could be detected (Toubro *et al.*,1995). Nevertheless, there is accumulating evidence that a low magnitude of one or more of these components of EE is involved in the aetiology of obesity, but the mechanisms responsible remain obscure.

LOW METABOLIC RATE AS A RISK FACTOR

Prospective studies

A low relative REE, expressed in relation to fat-free mass, has been found to be a risk factor for subsequent weight gain. In a prospective study in Pima Indians, Ravussin *et al.* (1988) demonstrated that both a low relative REE and a low relative 24-hour EE were risk factors for body weight gain. After 4 years of follow-up, the risk of gaining 10 kg was approximately seven times greater in those subjects with the lowest relative REE (lower tertile) than in those with the highest REE (higher tertile). Relative 24-hour EE was estimated to be responsible for up to 40% of the weight change.

Studies in Caucasian children have produced concordant results. In a study of EE in free-living infants born to lean and obese mothers, none of the infants born to lean mothers became obese in the first year of life, whereas 50% of the infants born to the overweight mothers became obese (Roberts *et al.*, 1988). The total EE of the infants who later became obese was 20% lower than that of the other groups. The shortcoming of this study is that only six overweight infants were studied, and only three of these remained overweight at 1 year of age. In another study of children 4–5 years old, Griffiths *et al.* (1990) reported that the REE and estimated total EE of those with an obese parent was 16% and 22% lower, respectively, than that of children whose parents had never been obese.

Studies on formerly obese subjects

To study the interaction between nutrient intake and metabolism in obese subjects in a search for the causes of obesity may be misguided, since energy expenditure, substrate utilization and regulatory hormones and substrates are all altered as a result of changes in body size and composition. This is the classic shortcoming of cross-sectional and case–control studies. Another approach to studying the possible role of low EE in the development of obesity is to study formerly obese subjects, assuming that their EE reverts to its preobese condition after weight normalization. The results obtained from such studies, comparing normal-weight, formerly obese, individuals (post-obese) with matched controls without a weight problem history are at first hand much easier to interpret (despite the difficulties involved in maintaining a weight stable state in post-obese subjects). A low relative REE and 24-hour EE have been found in some, but not all, formerly obese subjects, and the somewhat conflicting results can, at least partly, be explained by the selection of post-obese subjects, experimental conditions and lack of statistical power.

In the classic study of post-obese women by Geissler *et al.* (1987) it was found that, at three different levels of physical activity, the post-obese had a 15% lower 24-hour EE than matched controls. This study has been criticized for a poorly controlled activity programme, but a later reanalysis found that basal metabolic rate was 10% lower, and thermogenesis 50% lower, in the post-obese subjects than in the matched controls (Shah *et al.*, 1988). When taking the lower FFM into account, the group difference tended to vanish, though the relative EE remained slightly lower in the post-obese group.

After taking differences in FFM into account, Bukkens *et al.* (1991) reported a non-significant 5% lower REE in six post-obese individuals as compared with controls. McNeill *et al.* (1990) measured 24-hour EE and REE in six post-obese women and in matched controls and found a non-significant 7% lower 24-hour EE in the post-obese group. Goldberg *et al.* (1991) measured total free-living EE in post-obese and matched controls by doubly labelled water, and 24-hour EE in a respiratory chamber. They found no difference in EE, independently of method and way of expressing the data. Recently, a study with larger groups (18 post-obese and 14 controls) found that REE was 1317 kcal day^{-1} and 1341 kcal day^{-1} in post-obese and controls respectively (Amatruda *et al.*, 1993).

It is doubtful whether these studies possess the statistical power to disclose whether REE was lower in post-obese individuals and if the subnormal EE was present in the majority of cases. According to Ravussin *et al.* (1988) a low REE is not the cause of obesity, but rather a risk factor for weight gain and obesity. If the data on REE from these selected studies were pooled, however, it would probably become apparent that a higher proportion of the post-obese subjects exhibited a REE below the value predicted from FFM and FM.

A total of 28 post-obese women and a similar number of controls were assessed in a recent reanalysis that pooled data on REE from six studies in post-obese and matched controls. Age, body weight and composition were similar in the two groups (FFM 46.4 versus 46.7 kg). In this cohort REE was found to be 8% lower in the post-obese group ($P < 0.02$). Free T$_3$ concentration was 30% lower ($P < 0.01$) and plasma androstendione concentration marginally lower ($P = 0.07$) in the post-obese group than in controls. Adjustments for differences in FFM, FM and plasma androstendione did not influence the difference in REE, while adjustment for free T$_3$ concentrations eliminated the difference. This observation, however, does not prove that the lower REE of post-obese women is due to a lower thyroid hormone activity, but it certainly warrants more study.

In conclusion, a low REE for a given body composition is a risk factor for weight gain and obesity, and a low REE is found more frequently among formerly obese individuals, who may be presumed to have a genetic predisposition to obesity, than in a control group.

THE EFFECT OF DIETARY FAT/CARBOHYDRATE ON ENERGY EXPENDITURE

The inconsistency of the result on REE among post-obese groups may be partly explained by differences in the diets consumed during and preceding the measurement. Lean and James (1988) compared 24-hour EE and substrate utilization in obese, post-obese and normal-weight women. They were studied while in precise energy balance and consuming two iso-energetic diets, a low-fat diet (3% energy as fat, 82% carbohydrate) and a high-fat diet (40% fat and 45% carbohydrate). In addition, they were studied with the same high-fat diet supplemented with carbohydrate to 150% of energy balance (Lean *et al.*, 1988). Multiple regression analysis showed a linear relation between carbohydrate intake and 24-hour EE. There was a significant positive slope in the post-obese group, while the 24-hour EE was constant and unrelated to dietary carbohydrate intake in the control group. On the high-carbohydrate diet 24-hour EE was significantly higher in the post-obese group than in the control group, while 24-hour EE was lower in the post-obese group on the high-fat diet. These results demonstrate that post-obese and normal controls respond differently to changes in dietary carbohydrate content.

Furthermore, SNS reactivity may be subject to a similar high sensitivity to dietary carbohydrate, resulting in increased activity during high-carbohydrate feeding and reduced activity during low-carbohydrate (high-fat) feeding. We studied post-obese women who had been weight stable for at least 7 weeks, and compared them with controls matched with respect to age, height, weight and body composition (Astrup *et al.*, 1992b). On a standardized diet providing 30% energy from fat, 55% from carbohydrate and 15% from protein, 24-hour EE was 8% higher in the post-obese than in the controls. The difference was present both during sleep and in the day-time. Plasma noradrenaline concentration was increased by 50% in the post-obese as compared with the control group, and in a multiple regression analysis noradrenaline levels accounted for 65% of the variance in 24-hour EE and explained the entire difference between the two groups (Astrup *et al.*, 1992b). These results confirm those reported by Lean and James (1988) and Lean *et al.* (1988), except that our post-obese subjects were responsive to a diet containing less carbohydrate than reported in their study. In a subsequent study we established a dose–response relation between dietary carbohydrate content and 24-hour EE in post-obese women, while no such relation could be established in controls (Figure 3.1) (Astrup *et al.*, 1994).

In this study the increase in dietary carbohydrate content produced increases in free T_3 index, plasma noradrenaline (Figure 3.2), and androstendione concentrations, which together could explain the concomitant increase in 24-hour EE. This different responsiveness of REE of post-obese and control subjects to carbohydrates may be due to a genetic susceptibility

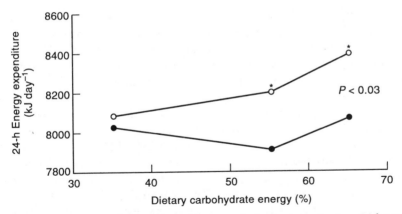

Figure 3.1 The effect of antecedent dietary carbohydrate content on 24-hour energy expenditure in post-obese women (○) and matched controls (●). The macronutrients were exchanged isoenergetically and the 35% and 65% carbohydrate diets were controlled for 5 days before the measurement. *Significantly different from 35% carbohydrate diet by ANOVA. Recalculated from Astrup *et al.* (1994)

of obesity-prone subjects. Alternatively, it may be that the high-carbohydrate diet must be consumed for a prolonged period before it increases EE. The successful post-obese subjects consumed a low-fat diet habitually, therefore perhaps responding more readily to a high-carbohydrate diet.

Although this issue has not been fully elucidated, there are some studies indicating that the carbohydrate content of the diet is also an important stimulator of energy expenditure in normal subjects. This line of evidence comes from a study comparing diet composition and resting metabolic rate (RMR) of vegetarians and non-vegetarians (Toth and Poehlman, 1994).

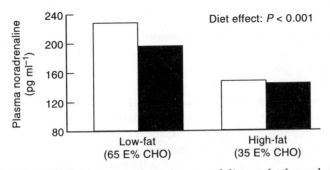

Figure 3.2 The effect of isoenergetic exchanges of dietary fat for carbohydrate on fasting venous plasma noradrenaline concentration in post-obese women (□) and matched controls (■). Diet effect, $P < 0.001$; group effect, NS; and diet × group, NS (Astrup *et al.*, 1994a). E, dietary energy.

Vegetarians reported a greater intake of carbohydrates than non-vegetarians (62% versus 51% food energy), whereas no difference was found in total energy intake, body composition or aerobic capacity. Vegetarians exhibited an 11% higher RMR, which could be explained by their higher SNS activity due to the higher carbohydrate intake.

Dietary intervention studies also support the hypothesis that a high-carbohydrate diet increases EE. Despite a weight loss during 20 weeks on an *ad libitum* low-fat, high-carbohydrate diet, energy intake increased by 19% compared with a control group consuming a high-fat diet (Prewitt *et al.*, 1991). An analysis of physical activity level could not disclose any change in daily activity level, which suggests that other components of energy expenditure were affected. The reason that some studies in non-obese and obese subjects have failed to detect any effect of diet composition on 24-hour EE may be that they have generally measured 24-hour EE after only a few days' exposure to the high-carbohydrate diet.

OXIDATIVE AUTOREGULATION

It was generally accepted, until recently, that the body is 'energy blind', i.e. that each individual has an oxidative autoregulation that is capable of rapid adjustments, altering the relative oxidation of fat and carbohydrates to match changes in dietary composition. Obviously, the achievement of macronutrient balance requires that the net oxidation of each nutrient equals the average composition of the macronutrients in the diet. Thus, increasing the fat content in the diet requires a matching increase in the oxidation of fat (Flatt, 1988,1989; Astrup and Raben, 1992).

There seems, however, to be differences between individuals as to how readily their autoregulation increases fat oxidation to match intake when challenged with a high-fat diet (Astrup *et al.*, 1994a). A significant part of these inter-individual differences may have a genetic background, although acquired disorders are certainly still possibilities, e.g. smoking cessation or treatment with obesity-promoting drugs such as sodium valproate. In subjects predisposed to obesity, a dysfunction of their autoregulation leads to an insufficient fat oxidation when challenged with a high-fat diet, which promotes enlargement of fat stores. This is a self-limiting process, because an increase in body fat stores will increase fat oxidation through an elevated level of circulating free fatty acids, which in turn increases substrate supply and hence stimulates oxidation (Schutz *et al.*, 1992). One may therefore regard obesity as a compensatory mechanism by which the body increases its fat oxidation to match the amount ingested in a high-fat diet (Astrup *et al.*, 1994a). Notably, the positive fat balance emerges, at least partly, from an excessive energy intake.

The time required to achieve balance for each macronutrient varies as a function of the amount ingested each day in relation to the total stores of that nutrient. A low-fat/high-carbohydrate diet is less likely to produce obesity than a high-fat diet because of the limited capacity of the body to store carbohydrate as glycogen. Net lipogenesis, i.e. the conversion of carbohydrate to lipid, is energetically an expensive transformation, which does not normally take place in the human species (Acheson *et al.*, 1984; Hellerstein *et al.*, 1991). Neurohumoral mediators, released as a function of sizes of the glycogen stores, are probably the link between macronutrient stores and energy intake. When the glycogen stores are filled, afferent signals to the brain will promote satiety. By contrast, body fat stores are much larger in relation to the daily fat intake, implying an almost unlimited capacity for fat storage.

An impaired fat metabolism in obesity-prone individuals

Evidence indicates that a combination of deficient fat oxidation and enhanced fat deposition exists (i.e. altered nutrient partitioning) in subjects with the predisposition to obesity. In a prospective study, 24-hour RQ was measured at baseline in Pima Indians fed a controlled diet, and it was found that those with a high RQ (low ratio of fat to carbohydrate oxidation) were at 2.5 times greater risk of a weight gain of 5 kg than those with a low RQ (Zurlo *et al.*, 1990b).

Studies in the post-obese also support the concept that fat oxidation may be impaired in predisposed subjects. Lean and James (1988) and Lean *et al.* (1988) reported striking differences in substrate handling by the obese, post-obese and controls. While mean 24-hour RQ was similar in the obese and in the control group, it was significantly higher in the post-obese group, during both fasting and the high-fat-diet. This indicates that the post-obese group utilized relatively less fat and relatively more carbohydrate than the control group during fasting and on the high-fat days.

We have tested the ability of post-obese women to adjust macronutrient oxidation in response to three isocaloric diets – a low-fat (20%), a medium-fat (30%) and a high-fat diet (50% fat energy) – using 24-hour calorimetry (Astrup *et al.*, 1994). No differences were found between groups on the low-fat and medium-fat diets. On the high-fat diet, however, the post-obese women failed to increase the ratio of fat to carbohydrate oxidation appropriately, which caused a positive fat balance. The preferential storage of fat in the post-obese group on the high-fat diet was caused by a failure to increase fat oxidation sufficiently to match the consumed fat. It is possible that the accompanying negative carbohydrate balance would tend to reduce glycogen stores, which is thought to be a signal for decreased satiety and increased hunger.

The phenomenon of an altered substrate pattern was also found after a high-fat meal (Raben *et al.*, 1994). Whereas the thermic effect of the meal was found to be similar in post-obese and control subjects, post-prandial fat oxidation was 2.5 times lower in the post-obese group. A similarly

suppressed concentration of plasma free fatty acid was seen post-pran-
dially in the post-obese subjects, possibly due to the more marked suppression of adrenaline and glucagon response found in this group (Andersen
et al., 1994). These findings demonstrate that the effect of a high-fat diet on
fat balance is especially pronounced in susceptible individuals, in whom
weight gain may eventually progress to obesity.

DIET COMPOSITION AND OBESITY

There is reliable evidence that obese subjects habitually consume a diet
with a higher fat content than normal-weight subjects. This could be the
mechanism that precipitates the expression of a genetic tendency, causes
a reduction in energy expenditure, and stimulates appetite via an impaired
post-prandial fat oxidation. It is, therefore, of interest to assess cross-sectional and longitudinal studies that have examined the relationship between dietary fat/carbohydrate and body fatness.

Cross-sectional and case–control studies

Most studies have examined the relation between intake of total carbohydrates, expressed in energy-%, and body fatness. Only four studies are
left for consideration (Tucker and Kano, 1992) if the studies lacking the
required positive association between body fatness and 24-hour energy
intake are excluded (Fehily *et al.*, 1984; Dreon *et al.*, 1988; Romieu *et al.*, 1989;
Miller *et al.*, 1990; Johannsson *et al.*, 1992; Lewis *et al.*, 1992; Slattery *et al.*,
1992). These four studies are in agreement, and demonstrate an inverse
relation between carbohydrate energy-% and body weight. Nevertheless,
the majority of the excluded studies also demonstrate an inverse relation
between energy-% carbohydrate and body weight, which supports the idea
that it is dietary fat intake that is most severely under-reported.

If studies relating sugars to body weight are assessed by the same criteria, then only two studies pass for consideration. They both demonstrate
that sucrose energy-% is negatively related to fatness (Tremblay *et al.*, 1989;
Bolton-Smith and Woodward, 1994). Bolton-Smith and Woodward (1994),
for example, stratified the population into percentiles according to sucrose
energy-% and found the lowest prevalence of obesity among those who
had the highest dietary sucrose content.

In the valid cross-sectional studies, case–control analysis of dietary composition in obese versus non-obese subjects consistently showed that obese
individuals consume a diet with a higher fat and a lower carbohydrate
content than non-obese. The diet of the obese groups has been found to be
5–8 fat energy-% higher than in the control groups (Table 3.1).

Miller *et al.* (1990) found that sugars accounted for 15.1% of consumed
energy in obese women, compared with 20.7% in the lean control group

Table 3.1 Case–control analysis of fat energy-% in obese subjects and controls

Study group	Energy-%		Fat mass (kg) (body weight)	Reference
	Fat	Carbohydrate		
Obese females	36	44 (15)	39 (90 kg)	Miller *et al.* (1990)
Lean females	29	53 (21)	9 (53 kg)	Miller *et al.* (1990)
Obese females	43	42	– (83 kg)	Tucker and Kano (1992)
Lean females	38	46	– (56 kg)	Tucker and Kano (1992)
Obese boys	39	49	16 (51 kg)	Gazzaniga *et al.* (1993)
Non-obese boys	31	55	4 (34 kg)	Gazzaniga *et al.* (1993)
Obese girls	39	49	19 (58 kg)	Gazzaniga *et al.* (1993)
Non-obese girls	34	53	6 (35 kg)	Gazzaniga *et al.* (1993)

(Gazzaniga *et al.*, 1993). A similar, but non-significant, trend was found in males (Gazzaniga *et al.*, 1993). Clearly, there is a need for a biological marker of habitual macronutrient intake. A proxy for dietary macronutrient composition can be obtained indirectly by measurement of substrate oxidations, because the oxidative pattern seems to be relatively undisturbed by changes in dietary fat content in the first 24 hours. Using 24-hour calorimetry Astrup *et al.* (1994b, c) found oxidative fat energy in overweight and obese subjects to be higher than in normal-weight controls (40.2% versus 36.0%, $P<0.02$). Unfortunately this method only provides information about total fat and carbohydrate intakes.

Longitudinal studies

The few valid longitudinal studies addressing the relation between dietary composition and body fatness suggest that dietary fat content is positively, and total carbohydrate content negatively, associated to subsequent weight gain (Eck *et al.*, 1992; Klesges *et al.*, 1992; Heitmann *et al.*, 1995). None of the valid studies, however, provide information about sugars. Interestingly, in The Nurses' Health Study, the strongest risk factor for subsequent weight gain was intake of saccharin (Colditz *et al.*, 1990). Unfortunately, the validity of this study is limited by the marked under-reporting of energy intake. A cross-sectional study has also observed higher intakes of high-intensity sweeteners among obese subjects (Lincoln, 1972), and another longitudinal study has reported that a high intake of high-intensity sweeteners is associated with prospective weight gain (Stellman and Garfinkel, 1988). These studies do not, however, prove a causal relationship between the replacement of sugars with high-intensity sweeteners and obesity, as high intakes may rather be a marker linked to the behaviour and lifestyle of obese individuals. Nevertheless, they indicate that even a substantial replacement of sugars by high-intensity sweeteners is insufficient to prevent weight gain and obesity in susceptible individuals.

Taste preferences in obesity

The selection of a diet with a higher fat content may be due to obesity-related specific taste preferences. Drewnowski *et al.* (1985) reported that, compared with normal-weight subjects, obese subjects exhibited enhanced preferences for high-fat contents in a sweetened, milk-based test system. More recently, Mela and Sacchetti (1991) examined sensory preferences by testing with different fat-containing foods. They found a positive correlation between overall fat preference and per cent body fat.

CONCLUSION

There is accumulating evidence to support the suggestion that dietary fat–carbohydrate ratio is important in the regulation of energy balance. The ratio has a substantial impact on *ad libitum* energy intake, and obesity-prone individuals may possess an enhanced susceptibility owing to a deficient fat oxidative autoregulation. The carbohydrate content of the diet regulates SNS activity and has an effect on energy expenditure that is more marked in obesity-prone subjects. Consequently, reducing the dietary fat–carbohydrate ratio promotes satiety and reduces energy intake, increases energy expenditure and causes spontaneous weight loss in obese patients, even when the diet is consumed *ad libitum* (Sheppard *et al.*, 1991; Schlundt *et al.*, 1993). An increased preference for high-fat foods has been found in obese subjects, and it is possible that this may be the reason why obese individuals generally consume a diet with a higher fat content than matched controls.

REFERENCES

Acheson K, Schutz Y, Bessard T *et al.* (1984). Nutritional influence on lipogenesis and thermogenesis after a carbohydrate meal. *American Journal of Physiology* **246**: E62–E70.

Amatruda J M, Statt M C, Welle S L (1993). Total and resting energy expenditure in obese women reduced to ideal body weight. *Journal of Clinical Investigation* **92**: 1236–1242.

Andersen H B, Raben A, Astrup A, Christensen N J (1994). Plasma adrenaline concentration is lower in post-obese than in never obese women in the basal state, in response to sham-feeding and after food intake. *Clinical Science* **87**: 69–74.

Astrup A, Raben A (1992). Obesity: an inherited metabolic deficiency in the control of macronutrient balance? *European Journal of Clinical Nutrition* **46**: 611–620.

Astrup A, Buemann B, Christensen N J, Madsen J (1992a). 24-hour energy expenditure and sympathetic activity in post-obese women consuming a high-carbohydrate diet. *American Journal of Physiology* **262**: E282–E288.

Astrup A, Buemann B, Christensen N J et al. (1992b). The contribution of body composition, substrates and hormones to the variability in energy expenditure and substrate utilization in pre-menopausal women. *Journal of Clinical Endocrinology and Metabolism* **74**: 279–286.

Astrup A, Buemann B, Christensen N J, Toubro S (1994a). Failure to increase lipid oxidation in response to increasing dietary fat content in formerly obese women. *American Journal of Physiology* **266**: E592-E599.

Astrup A, Buemann B, Western P et al. (1994b). Obesity as an adaptation to a high-fat diet: evidence from a cross-sectional study. *American Journal of Clinical Nutrition* **59**: 350–355.

Astrup A, Western P, Toubro S, Raben A, Buemann B, Christensen N J (1994c). Obesity as an adaptation to a high-fat diet. Reply to AM Prentice et al. *American Journal of Clinical Nutrition* **60**: 641–642.

Bogardus C, Lillioja S, Ravussin E et al. (1986). Familial dependence of resting metabolic rate. *New England Journal of Medicine* **315**: 96–100.

Bolton-Smith C, Woodward M (1994). The prevalence of overweight and obesity in different fat and sugar consumption groups. *International Journal of Obesity* **18**: 820–828.

Bouchard C, Tremblay A, Nadeau A et al. (1989). Genetic effect in resting and exercise metabolic rates. *Metabolism* **38**: 364–370.

Bukkens S G F, McNeill G, Smith J S, Morrison D C (1991). Postprandial thermogenesis in post-obese women and weight-matched controls. *International Journal of Obesity* **15**: 147–154.

Colditz G A, Willett W C, Stampfer M J, London S J, Segal M R, Speizer F E (1990). Patterns of weight change and their relation to diet in a cohort of healthy women. *American Journal of Clinical Nutrition* **51**: 1100–1105.

Dreon D M, Frey-Hewitt B, Ellsworth N et al. (1988). Dietary fat:carbohydrate ratio and obesity in middle-aged men. *American Journal of Clinical Nutrition* **47**: 995–1000.

Drewnowski A, Brunzell J D, Sande K et al. (1985). Sweet tooth reconsidered: taste preferences in human obesity. *Physiology and Behaviour* **35**: 617–622.

Eck L H, Klesges R C, Hanson C L, Slawson D (1992). Children at familial risk for obesity: an examination of dietary intake, physical activity and weight status. *International Journal of Obesity* **16**: 71–78.

Fehily A M, Phillips K M, Yarnell J W G (1984). Diet, smoking, social class, and BMI in the Caerphilly Heart Disease Study. *American Journal of Clinical Nutrition* **40**: 827–833.

Flatt J P (1988). Importance of nutrient balance in body weight regulation. *Diabetes Metabolism Reviews* **6**: 571–581.

Flatt J P (1989). Differences in the regulation of carbohydrate and fat metabolism and their implications for body weight maintenance. In: Lardy H, Stratman F (eds) *Hormones, Thermogenesis and Obesity.* Elsevier, New York, pp. 3–18.

Gazzaniga J M, Burns R D, Burns T L (1993). The relationship between diet composition and body fatness, with adjustment for resting energy expenditure and physical activity in preadolescent children. *American Journal of Clinical Nutrition* **58**: 21–28.

Geissler C A, Miller D S, Shah M (1987). The daily metabolic rate of the post-obese and the lean. *American Journal of Clinical Nutrition* **45**: 914–920.

Goldberg G R, Black A E, Prentice A M, Coward W A (1991). No evidence of lower energy expenditure in post-obese women. *Proceedings of the Nutrition Society* **50**: 109A.

Griffiths M, Payne P R, Stunkard A J *et al.* (1990). Metabolic rate and physical development in children at risk of obesity. *Lancet* **336**: 76–77.

Heitmann B L, Lissner L, Sørensen T I A, Bengtsson C (1995). Dietary fat intake promotes weight gain in predisposed individuals. A prospective population study of Swedish women. *International Journal of Obesity* **17**: 108.

Hellerstein M K, Christiansen M, Kaempler S *et al.* (1991). Measurement of *de novo* hepatic lipogenesis in humans using stable isotopes. *Journal of Clinical Investigation* **87**: 1841–1852.

Johansson I, Hallmans G, Asplund K (1992). Are risk factors for artherosclerosis in an area with a high incidence of cardiovascular disease related to diet? *Scandinavian Journal of Nutrition* **36**: 154–160.

Klesges R C, Klesges L M, Haddock C K, Eck L (1992). A longitudinal analysis of the impact of dietary intake and physical activity on weight change in adults. *American Journal of Clinical Nutrition* **55**: 818–822.

Lean M E J, James W P T (1988). Metabolic effects of isoenergetic nutrient exchange over 24 hours in relation to obesity in women. *International Journal of Obesity* **12**: 15–27.

Lean M E J, James WPT, Garthwaite P H (1988). Obesity without overeating? Reduced diet-induced thermogenesis in post-obese women, dependent on carbohydrate and not fat intake. In: Björntorp P, Rössner S (eds) *Obesity in Europe*. John Libbey, London. pp. 281–286.

Lewis C J, Park Y K, Dexter P B, Yetley E A (1992). Nutrient intakes and body weights of persons consuming high and moderate levels of added sugars. *Journal of the American Dietetic Association* **92**: 708.

Lincoln J E (1972). Calorie intake, obesity, and physical activity. *American Journal of Clinical Nutrition* **25**: 390.

McNeill G, Bukkens S G F, Morrison D C, Smith J S (1990). Energy intake and energy expenditure in post-obese women and weight-matched controls. *Proceedings of the Nutrition Society* **49**: 14A.

Mela D J, Sacchetti D A (1991). Sensory preferences for fats: relationships with diet and body composition. *American Journal of Clinical Nutrition* **53**: 908–915.

Miller W C, Lindeman A K, Wallace J, Niederpruem M (1990). Diet composition, energy intake, and exercise in relation to body fat in men and women. *American Journal of Clinical Nutrition* **52**: 426–430.

Poehlman E T, Melby C L, Bradylak S J (1988). Resting metabolic rate and postprandial thermogenesis in highly trained and untrained males. *American Journal of Physiology* **47**: 793–798.

Prewitt T E, Schmeisser D, Bowen P E *et al.* (1991). Changes in body weight, body composition, and energy intake in women fed high- and low-fat diets. *American Journal of Clinical Nutrition* **54**: 304–310.

Raben A, Andersen H B, Christensen N J *et al.* (1994). Evidence for an abnormal postprandial response to a high-fat meal in women predisposed to obesity. *American Journal of Physiology* **267**: E549–E559.

Ravussin E, Bogardus C (1989). Relationship of genetics, age, and physical fitness to daily energy expenditure and fuel utilization. *American Journal of Clinical Nutrition* **49**: 968–975.

Ravussin E, Lillioja S, Knowler WC *et al.* (1988). Reduced rate of energy expenditure as a risk factor for body-weight gain. *New England Journal of Medicine* **318**: 467–472.

Rising R, Keys A, Ravussin E, Bogardus C (1992). Concomitant interindividual variation in body temperature and metabolic rate. *American Journal of Physiology* **263**: E730–E734.

Roberts S B, Savage J, Coward W A *et al.* (1988). Energy expenditure and intake in infants born to lean and overweight mothers. *New England Journal of Medicine* **318**: 461–6.

Romieu I, Walter C W, Stampfer M J *et al.* (1989). Energy intake and other determinants of relative weight. *American Journal of Clinical Nutrition* **47**: 406–412.

Saad M F, Alger S A, Zurlo F *et al.* (1991). Ethnic differences in sympathetic nervous system-mediated energy expenditure. *American Journal of Physiology* **261**: E789–E794.

Schlundt D G, Hill J O, Pope-Cordle J *et al.* (1993). Randomised evaluation of a low fat *ad libitum* carbohydrate diet for weight reduction. *International Journal of Obesity* **17**: 623–629.

Schutz Y, Tremblay A, Weinsier R L, Nelson K M (1992). Role of fat oxidation in the long-term stabilization of body weight in obese women. *American Journal of Clinical Nutrition* **55**: 670–674.

Shah M, Miller D S, Geissler C A (1988). Lower metabolic rates of post-obese versus lean women: thermogenesis, basal metabolic rate and genetics. *European Journal of Clinical Nutrition* **42**: 741–752.

Sheppard L, Kristal A R, Kushi L H (1991). Weight loss in women participating in a randomised trial of low-fat diets. *American Journal of Clinical Nutrition* **54**: 821–828.

Slattery M L, McDonald A, Bild D E *et al.* (1992). Associations of body fat and its distribution with dietary intake, physical activity, alcohol, and smoking in blacks and whites. *American Journal of Clinical Nutrition* **55**: 943–949.

Spraul M, Ravussin E, Fontvielle A M *et al.* (1993). Reduced sympathetic nervous activity. A potential mechanism predisposing to body weight gain. *Journal of Clinical Investigation* **92**: 1730–1735.

Stellman S D, Garfinkel L (1988). Patterns of artificial sweetener use and weight change in an American cancer society prospective study. *Appetite* **11**: 85.

Svendsen O L, Hassager C, Christiansen C (1993). Impact of regional and total body composition and hormones on resting energy expenditure in overweight post-menopausal women. *Metabolism* **42**: 1588–1591.

Toth M J, Poehlman E T (1994). Sympathetic nervous system activity and resting metabolic rate in vegetarians. *Metabolism* **43**: 621–625.

Toubro S, Sørensen T I A, Christensen N J, Astrup A (1995). Sibling resemblance of determinants of 24-hour energy expenditure. The importance of thyroid status and sympathetic activity. *Journal of Clinical Investigation* (in press).

Tremblay A, Plourde G, Despres J-P, Bouchard C (1989). Impact of dietary fat content and fat oxidation on energy intake in humans. *American Journal of Clinical Nutrition* **49**: 799–805.

Tucker L A, Kano M J (1992). Dietary fat and body fat: a multivariate study of 205 adult females. *American Journal of Clinical Nutrition* **56**: 616–622.

Zurlo F, Larson K, Bogardus C, Ravussin E (1990a). Skeletal muscle metabolism is a major determinant of resting energy expenditure. *Journal of Clinical Investigation* **86**: 1423–1427.

Zurlo F, Lillioja S, Puente A E D *et al.* (1990b). Low ratio of fat to carbohydrate oxidation as a predictor of weight gain: study of 24-hour RQ. *American Journal of Physiology* **22**: E650–E657.

CHAPTER 4

Metabolic response to slimming

Susan A. Jebb

INTRODUCTION

In the last decade the prevalence of obesity (BMI > 30 kg m^{-2}) in Britain has doubled (Gregory *et al.*, 1990). At the same time the diet industry is also getting bigger. By 1994 the sales of meal replacement products had exceeded £80 million and over £5 million was spent on slimming magazines (West, 1994). It seems that more and more time and money is being spent on ways and means to lose weight. Combining these observations suggests that weight loss is not nearly as easy as weight gain.

The reasons for this may be considered to be physiological or psychological, but there is also a great deal of interplay between these two aspects. Deeply held beliefs about the physiology of slimming undoubtedly contribute to the state of mind of dieters. 'It's my metabolism' is often given as the socially acceptable justification for obesity, which goes some way towards attracting the sort of sympathy reserved for those with an illness and rarely given to those with what is perceived to be a self-inflicted problem. The phrase 'Dieting makes you fat' sums up the impressions of a generation who have tried and failed to lose weight and who now take some comfort in the fact that their metabolism is against them. There is an increasing wave of scepticism for the latest diet from those who feel that attempts at weight control may be futile. But how justified is the fear that the metabolic response to slimming is an insurmountable barrier to successful weight loss?

Although most dieters strive to lose some of their body fat, this is popularly interpreted as a desire to lose weight. Changes in body energy stores are measured as changes in body weight, which is used as a proxy for fat loss. For this to occur requires a period of net negative energy balance. This

Weight Control
Edited by Richard Cottrell.
Published in 1995 by Chapman & Hall, London. ISBN 0 412 73600 4

will follow a period of weight gain, and associated positive energy balance, or at best energy homeostasis, so it is perhaps almost inevitable that the imposition of a state of negative energy balance will initiate a series of physiological responses in terms of energy intake, expenditure and body composition. This chapter will consider some of the factors that determine the nature of this metabolic response.

SHORT-TERM CONSEQUENCES OF SLIMMING

Energy intake

Energy intake is probably the variable in the energy balance equation that offers the individual the greatest opportunity for control. Few weight loss programmes will succeed without a sustained reduction in energy intake. However, we have little understanding of the ways in which the hunger drive to maintain energy intake is affected by a sustained effort to eat less. Certainly this is a powerful effect, and there are many reports of the association between energy restriction and subsequent binge eating (Russell, 1987). This is an area of considerable current research.

Energy expenditure

Changes in resting energy expenditure (REE)

After more than a few days, energy restriction causes a decrease in basal energy expenditure, although this effect may be attenuated by exercise or specific pharmacological agents. However, in the very first few days of total starvation there is often a small absolute increase in basal metabolic rate (BMR) relative to values obtained after an overnight fast. This may be due to a number of metabolic processes, including increased gluconeogenesis, triglyceride–fatty acid cycling, protein–amino acid cycling and acetyl CoA–ketone cycling (Elia, 1992).

The subsequent decrease in BMR occurs in both lean and obese subjects. In one study in which three lean young men were underfed on a diet of 3.5 MJ per day for 12 days within a whole-body calorimeter, BMR decreased by a mean of 15% while body weight decreased by only 4% (Parkinson, 1990).

There are a large number of studies in which the decrease in BMR has been measured during dieting. Figure 4.1 represents data from 515 subjects in 29 published studies of diets lasting from 1 to 26 weeks (Prentice *et al.*, 1991). In spite of the variation between studies, the decrease in BMR over the period of dieting is generally between 5% and 25%.

Some of the variability may be explained by differences in the diet regimen used in the various studies, which ranged from very low-calorie diets (VLCDs), providing less than 500 kcal per day to only mild energy

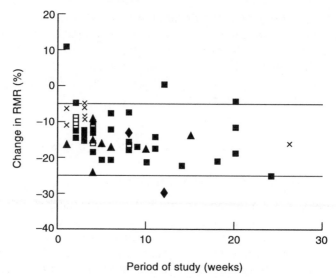

Period of study (weeks)

Figure 4.1 Suppression of metabolic rate (BMR or RMR) reported from 515 subjects (both sexes) in 29 studies of weight loss employing a variety of diets and lasting from 1 to 26 weeks. Each point represents a group mean. Data from Bray (1969), Apfelbaum *et al.* (1971), Rabast *et al.* (1981), Dore *et al.* (1982), Bessard *et al.* (1983), Webb and Abrams (1983), Schutz *et al.* (1984), de-Boer *et al.* (1986), Finer *et al.* (1986), Welle and Campbell (1986), Barrows and Snook (1987), Belko *et al.* (1987), Henson *et al.* (1987), Hill *et al.* (1987), Garby *et al.* (1988), Hendler and Bonde (1988), Phinney *et al.* (1988), Poole and Henson (1988), Alban-Davies *et al.* (1989), Coxon *et al.* (1989), de-Groot *et al.* (1989), Elliot *et al.* (1989), Garrow and Webster (1989), Hainer *et al.* (1989), Heymsfield *et al.* (1989), Rattan *et al.* (1989); Foster *et al.* (1990), van Dale *et al.* (1990a, b). Reproduced from Prentice *et al.* (1991) The physiological response to slimming. *Proceedings of the Nutrition Society*, **50**: 441–448, with permission of Cambridge University Press.

restriction. If the data are re-expressed in relation to the weight lost, the response seems more consistent and appears to plateau at around –20% to –25% of initial RMR, in those who have lost in excess of 20% of their initial body weight (Figure 4.2). This figure highlights a few studies in which lean individuals have undergone a period of energy restriction. The data are largely consistent with those from obese subjects with the notable exception of Keys *et al.* (1950). The Keys data are taken from the now classic studies of semistarvation. During the Second World War a group of conscientious objectors who were not initially overweight were underfed for 26 weeks, by which stage they had lost up to 25% of their initial body weight and the final decrease in BMR approached 40%.

The rate of weight loss may also be important in terms of the suppression of RMR, but few studies have directly addressed this issue. An exception is that of Foster *et al.* (1990), who compared two slimming regimens. The first provided 1200 kcal per day for 24 weeks, while the second included a 7-week period of only 500 kcal per day within an otherwise similar regimen.

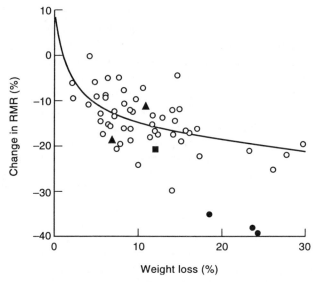

Figure 4.2 Suppression of BMR/RMR in relation to weight loss. Data from obese subjects as Figure 4.1 with exception of Welle and Campbell (1986), Coxon *et al.* (1989) and Rattan *et al.* (1989) in which percentage weight loss could not be calculated. Data from lean subjects taken from Jansen (1917) (■), Benedict *et al.* (1919) (▲), Keys *et al.* (1950) (●), Diaz *et al.* (1992) (○). Reproduced from Prentice *et al.* (1991) The physiological response to slimming. *Proceedings of the Nutrition Society*, **50**: 441–448, with permission of Cambridge University Press.

Although the time course of weight loss varied between the two groups, at the end of 24 weeks weight loss was surprisingly similar, suggesting an element of non-compliance. However, there were significant differences in RMR, which would also tend to reduce the magnitude of the energy difference between the two groups. In the VLCD group, RMR dropped by a maximum of 18% at week 10 and remained 11% lower at the end of the study, while in the group receiving 1200 kcal per day throughout RMR remained unchanged.

Further indirect evidence for a greater suppression of RMR during rapid weight loss, on highly restricted energy intakes, comes from the combined analysis of a number of studies. Figure 4.3 summarizes data for diets providing 400 kcal, 700 kcal and 1200 kcal per day. Predictably, those with the lowest energy intakes lost the greatest amount of weight, but there is also a significant difference in the degree of suppression of RMR. Diets of 700 kcal or less produce a decrease in RMR of greater than 15%, while those of 1200 kcal show a decrease of only 5%. This suggests that there may be a threshold of energy intake, perhaps around 1200 kcal per day, below which the perceived advantages of rapid weight loss may be offset by a greater suppression of energy expenditure.

However, this figure does not consider the changes in the suppression of energy expenditure with time. A study by de-Boer (1986) shows that energy expenditure within a whole-body calorimeter declines progressively during a VLCD, from a reduction of less than 5% by the end of day 1 to a nadir of 15% after 8 weeks. However, the decrease during dieting appears to be matched by an increase following cessation of the diet. What is perhaps most remarkable is the speed of the changes. One-third of the total decrease occurs after only 1 day and 6% is recovered the day after energy restriction ceases.

This post-diet increase in BMR is important, since the decrease in BMR during dieting has sometimes been interpreted as a permanent suppression of metabolic rate. Any lasting reduction in BMR would be of enormous consequence to dieters, who frequently report numerous dieting attempts within a year, let alone a lifetime. Evidence for the recovery of BMR after weight loss dates back to the work of Keys *et al.* (1950). After 26 weeks of underfeeding, the volunteers were refed on either a fast or a slow rehabilitation programme. In both cases BMR returned to prestarvation levels in parallel with the increase in body weight. More recently, BMR was measured in a group of obese women throughout three consecutive periods each comprising 2 weeks VLCD and 4 weeks *ad libitum* eating (Jebb *et al.*, 1991). After the full 18 weeks body weight had decreased by almost 6 kg but BMR was unchanged (Figure 4.4).

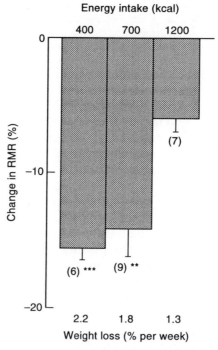

Figure 4.3 Suppression of BMR/RMR on diets providing different energy intakes 4–6 weeks after commencement of diet. Reproduced from Prentice *et al.* (1991) The physiological response to slimming. *Proceedings of the Nutrition Society*, **50**: 441–448, with permission of Cambridge University Press. **P < 0.01; ***P < 0.001.

Further evidence in support of the maintenance of metabolic rate comes from studies of the post-obese (otherwise known as successful slimmers), in whom RMR has been shown to be virtually identical to lean, never obese controls (Goldberg *et al.*, 1991). While these metabolic measurements cannot refute the remarkable propensity of individuals to regain lost weight, these data and those from the yo-yo dieting study suggest that this phenomenon cannot be attributed to metabolic changes in energy requirements.

Understanding the nature of the reduction in RMR during dieting might provide a rational basis for attenuating this effect. In part, the fall in BMR can be attributed to a decrease in FFM, and this forms the basis of the suggestion that exercise may prevent the fall in RMR. However, opinion is divided on this point.

A number of studies have compared changes in RMR in subjects following diet alone or diet plus exercise protocols (Figure 4.5). Although the majority show a protective benefit, with smaller decreases in RMR with exercise, the evidence is by no means overwhelming (Prentice *et al.*, 1991). Advocates of diet plus exercise claim that the failure to demonstrate a positive effect of exercise results from the failure to obtain the necessary exercise compliance. Sceptics respond with the observation that it is the difficulty of persuading obese people to exercise that will always be the limiting factor in the efficacy of this approach.

However, it is clear that changes in FFM do not account for all the decrease in BMR, and hormonal changes have been suggested as a further contributor.

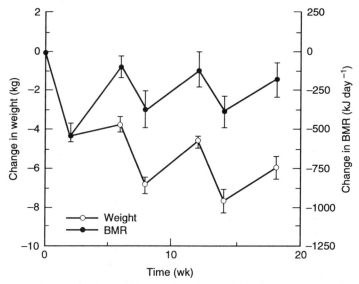

Figure 4.4 Changes in body weight and BMR during repeated periods of weight loss. Data from Prentice *et al.* (1991) The physiological response to slimming. *Proceedings of the Nutrition Society*, **50**: 441–448, with permission of Cambridge University Press.

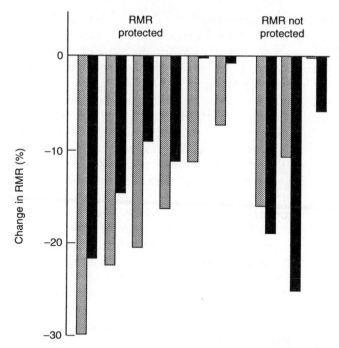

Figure 4.5 The effect of exercise on diet-induced reductions in RMR. Data from
Krotkiewski (1981), Belko *et al.* (1987), Hill *et al.* (1987), Phinney *et al.* (1988),
Heymsfield *et al.* (1989), Pavlou *et al.* (1989), van Dale *et al.* (1990a, b).
Reproduced from Prentice *et al.* (1991) The physiological response to slimming.
Proceedings of the Nutrition Society, **50**: 441–448, with permission of Cambridge
University Press.

Certainly part of the decrease in RMR may be mediated by a fall in circulating
free triiodothyronine, which commonly reaches 70% of prediet levels and in
some cases even as low as 50% (Prentice *et al.*, 1991). Additional measurements indicate that reverse T_3 shows a parallel rise, suggesting a change in
the conversion rate rather than altered release of thyroid hormones. Mean-
while T_4 remains unchanged. Not surprisingly, thyroid hormone adminis-
tration has been viewed as a potential therapeutic intervention. But, while
preventing the fall in RMR, it also produces an unacceptable rise in nitrogen
excretion and the loss of FFM. A study by Welle and Campbell (1986), in
which subjects received low-dose T_3 and T_4 (designed only to maintain
plasma levels within the physiological range), failed to abolish completely
the fall in RMR.

Changes in the sympathetic nervous system have also been documented,
but they do not correlate well with the change in RMR (Webber and
Macdonald, 1993). Other evidence suggests a reduction in sympathetic hormones in obese subjects during energy restriction and in patients with
anorexia nervosa (Landsberg and Young, 1983), but the relevance to the fall
in RMR is unclear.

Pharmacological interventions to stimulate metabolic rate, or at least alleviate the suppression caused by dieting, are an attractive option and have received considerable attention. A number of these, notably the β_3-agonists, have been developed to stimulate thermogenesis via a mechanism that is independent of those believed to be responsible for the physiological suppression of BMR. However, to date, there is no conventionally acceptable pharmacological agent, based on the stimulation of thermogenesis, officially licensed in Britain.

The physiological decrease in BMR during dieting is a real phenomenon, related both to the duration of dieting and to the magnitude of the energy deficit. BMR is only depressed by more than 20% after massive weight loss. It does not therefore preclude successful weight reduction and should not be invoked to account for difficulties in achieving weight loss. There is some evidence that VLCDs may exacerbate the reduction in BMR, while exercise probably has a protective effect. Perhaps most importantly of all, when dieting ceases metabolic rate returns to a level commensurate with the new body size.

Changes in total energy expenditure (TEE)

BMR is only part of the total energy requirement of an individual. Thermogenesis is also likely to be decreased, but since it is such a small component of total energy expenditure the potential for inducing change is small. However, changes in the energy cost of physical activity may be significant. With the development and application of the doubly labelled water technique it has become possible to measure total energy expenditure and, by difference from BMR, the energy cost of activity can be calculated (Prentice, 1988).

Exercise may exert a beneficial effect on weight loss not by reversing the adaptive decreases in RMR, but by increasing the physical activity component of total energy expenditure. In situations in which subjects choose to take part in a formal exercise programme this should perhaps be classified as a behavioural effect, rather than a metabolic consequence of slimming, but two recent studies have shown increases in the physical activity component of total energy expenditure in subjects who did not consciously undertake a formal exercise programme. The first is a study of four grossly obese patients with a mean weight of 136 kg (Fuller *et al.*, 1995). These patients had a gastroplasty operation in which the size of the stomach was reduced to less than 50 ml and as a consequence they lost over 40 kg or 30% of initial body weight (Table 4.1).

RMR decreased by 22% but TEE remained unchanged. In this case, spontaneous increases in physical activity were sufficient to counterbalance the decrease observed in RMR. These patients are of course an exceptional group in whom it might be argued that their initial weight restricted their physical activity and that weight reduction simply allowed them to adopt a more normal lifestyle and activity pattern. However, further evidence for

Table 4.1 Changes in energy metabolism following vertical banded gastroplasty (mean and SD)

	Before	After	Change (%)	
Weight (kg)	136.3 (24.3)	94.4 (13.6)	−30.7	$P < 0.001$
BMR (MJ day^{-1})	8.5 (0.7)	6.6 (0.2)	−22.4	$P < 0.01$
TEE (MJ day$^{-1)}$	11.9 (1.9)	12.4 (1.3)	+4.2	NS
Physical activity level (TEE/BMR)	1.4 (0.2)	1.9 (0.3)	+35.7	$P < 0.05$

(Data from Fuller *et al.* 1995).

the maintenance of TEE during weight reduction comes from a second study in subjects with BMIs ranging from 22 to 43 kg m^{-2} (Kreitzman *et al.*, 1993). A mean weight loss of 16 kg was achieved during a 10-week period on a VLCD. Overall REE decreased by 13%, most of which occurred in the first 3 weeks. During this time TEE was unchanged, suggesting an increase in physical activity that counterbalanced the physiological decrease in REE.

The cause of this increase in the energy cost of activity is unknown, and it is not clear that this effect is common to a wider group of dieters. However, it reinforces the difficulties of separating the metabolic, behavioural and psychological effects of slimming. Ultimately such divisions are academic since the dieting experience of an individual will represent the sum of metabolic plus behavioural effects and the way in which these phenomena are psychologically integrated by an individual trying to lose weight.

Body composition

For many dieters weight loss is often used as a proxy for fat loss, largely because it can be measured more easily and simply than body fat. However, obese subjects not only have more fat than their non-obese counterparts but more lean tissue too, in order to support the extra fat mass. It is therefore entirely appropriate that weight loss should comprise a mixture of both fat and FFM. If a 70-kg reference man with 12 kg of fat and 58 kg of FFM were to double his weight we might expect him to have 62 kg of fat and 78 kg of FFM (Elia, 1992).

FFM is a heterogeneous compartment of the body most simply accounting for the difference between total body weight and fat mass. It includes water, protein, glycogen, mineral and small quantities of other body constituents including free amino acids. There is a considerable amount of evidence that weight loss results in a decrease in each of these components, but what is appropriate loss and what is not?

To answer this question it is useful to consider the relationship between body fat and lean tissue. Forbes (1987) has proposed a model based on the observed body composition in women across a wide range of body weights.

This is a curvilinear relationship that becomes linear on log transformation (Figure 4.6). It is arguable that this figure is heavily influenced by the inclusion of a group of subjects with anorexia nervosa, but since this only affects those with very low levels of body fat mass we may otherwise assume that this represents the appropriate proportion of lean to fat tissue in healthy individuals.

The interpretation of this plot demonstrates that for an obese woman to lose 10 kg of fat she would also have to lose 2–3 kg of lean tissue in order to retain an appropriate body composition. However, as the initial body weight of the subjects decreases the loss of 10 kg fat would have to be associated with a progressively increasing quantity of lean tissue. This is, in itself, an important observation, since it suggests that the appropriate composition of weight loss will vary according to the initial amount of body fat.

If these data are replotted expressing the change in lean tissue as a ratio to the change in total body weight, it can be used as a standard to judge the appropriate composition of weight loss.

Figure 4.7 shows data from 548 subjects in whom the composition of weight loss was measured. These data suggest that the lean tissue component of weight lost on diets with a mild energy deficit, providing upwards of 1000 kcal per day, is equal to or less than the amount predicted from the Forbes model of normal body composition. However, diets that provide

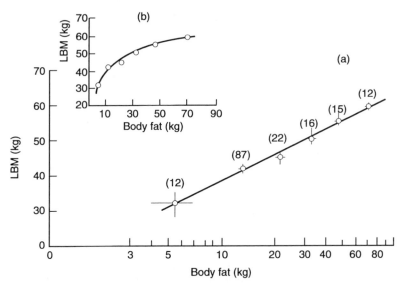

Figure 4.6 (a) Plot of lean body mass (LBM) versus $\log_{10}$ body fat for females grouped according to body fat content. Values are means with 2 SEM, represented by error bars, for numbers of subjects shown in parentheses. (b) Plot of LBM versus body fat from the same data. Reproduced from Forbes (1987) with permission.

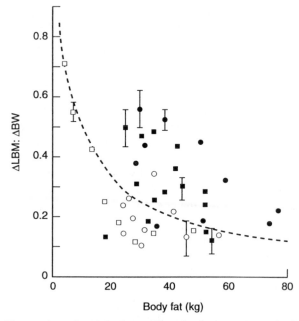

Figure 4.7   Proportion of weight lost as lean body mass in underfeeding experiments of at least 4 weeks' duration with subjects grouped according to midpoint body fat content and by energy intake. Reproduced from Prentice *et al.* (1991) The physiological response to slimming. *Proceedings of the Nutrition Society*, **50**: 441–448, with permission of Cambridge University Press. – – – line based on a relationship derived in Figure 4.6. ●, 0–400 kcal day⁻¹; ■, 500–900 kcal day⁻¹; ○, 1000–1400 kcal day⁻¹; □, 1500–1900 kcal day⁻¹.

progressively lower energy intakes tend to result in greater than expected losses of lean tissue. This seems to be particularly true of diets providing less than 400 kcal per day, in which case only 2 out of 10 studies show appropriate losses of lean tissue. Overall, this evidence suggests that the composition of weight loss is determined not only by initial body fat mass, but also by the energy deficit.

The strength of this model is that despite the heterogeneity of the sample and the use of a variety of methods to measure body composition there is still a striking relationship. Measuring body composition by indirect methods poses particular problems in patients losing weight, since many of the assumptions of the models may be violated, most notably losses of glycogen and changes in the hydration fraction of FFM.

A recent study has examined the metabolic effects of VLCDs using sophisticated multicompartment models to assess body composition changes during dieting (Ryde *et al.*, 1993). Subjects were asked to consume a diet containing only 405 kcal per day for 10 weeks. The mean proportion of weight lost as fat was 22%, with similar proportional losses of FFM in subjects in whom the initial BMI ranged from 22 to 43 kg m⁻² (Figure 4.8).

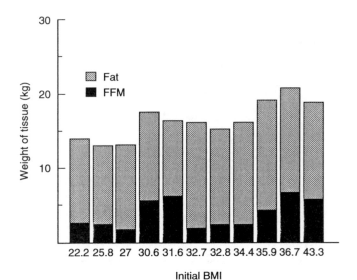

Figure 4.8 Individual composition of weight loss for subjects consuming 405 kcal for 10 weeks. Data from Ryde *et al.* (1993).

These data are entirely consistent with the Forbes model, showing appropriate losses of lean and fat tissue in individual subjects. Although it appears that the loss of lean tissue in subjects consuming a VLCD is less than would be expected, energy balance calculations using the measured total energy expenditure of individual subjects suggests that most subjects were consuming rather more than 400 kcal per day. The composition of weight loss therefore reflects what would be anticipated on a diet providing around 800 kcal per day.

Thus it seems that this study adds to the evidence in support of the Forbes model. However, in order to overcome residual errors in the interpretation of indirect body composition analysis, and to elucidate subtle differences in the composition of weight lost by lean and obese subjects, the most reliable studies are those in which lean tissue losses have been measured directly by nitrogen balance. Unfortunately, such data are few and far between.

Figure 4.9 shows daily nitrogen balance in groups of obese subjects receiving diets containing fewer than 800 kcal per day and 5–21 g of nitrogen. After initial nitrogen balance there is a large loss of nitrogen during the first week of dieting, which progressively reduces over the next few weeks, reaching a plateau after 3–4 weeks. The nitrogen loss during the first week is twofold greater than during the third or fourth week. This progressive reduction in the loss of nitrogen implies that the proportion of lean tissue lost becomes smaller with time.

Unfortunately, this conservation of lean tissue does not seem to be as effective for non-obese subjects during hypocaloric dieting or indeed total

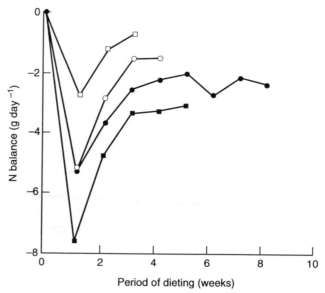

Figure 4.9 Daily nitrogen balance in groups of obese individuals during dieting. Data from Wilson and Lamberts (1979) (○), Hoffer *et al.* (1984) (●), Yang *et al.* (1981) (■), Hendler and Bonde, (1988) (□). Reproduced from Elia (1992) with permission.

starvation. Lean subjects, despite having a smaller FFM than their obese counterparts, maintain a higher daily nitrogen excretion. Figure 4.10 shows data from studies of total starvation in lean and obese subjects. The lean individuals were losing approximately 8–10 g of nitrogen per day or 50–60 g of protein throughout the period of starvation. In contrast, in the obese subjects, although the initial losses of nitrogen are similar to those in lean subjects, they quickly diminish, so that after only 10 days the losses of protein in the obese are approximately twofold lower than in lean subjects.

But few subjects choose to lose weight by total starvation. For those consuming hypocaloric diets there are important interactions between energy and protein in terms of overall nitrogen balance and the loss of lean tissue. When nitrogen intake is kept constant nitrogen balance is improved by increasing the energy intake. When energy intake is constant, nitrogen balance is improved by increasing the nitrogen intake, although there seems to be little effect above a threshold value of about 6–7 g of nitrogen per day. Thus, nitrogen losses can be minimized by diets providing in excess of about 40 g of protein per day and modest reductions in energy intake (Calloway and Spector, 1954).

These detailed nitrogen balance studies confirm the findings of the larger and more numerous studies of gross body composition by indirect methods, which together lead to a number of conclusions regarding the changes in body composition during slimming. Firstly, the composition of weight

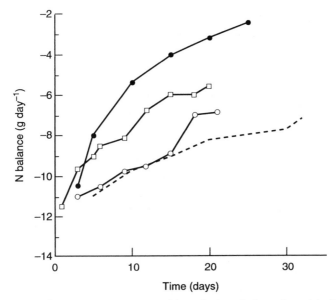

Figure 4.10 Daily nitrogen excretion of lean (....) and obese (——) individuals during total starvation. Data from Ballentyne (1973) (●), Young *et al.* (1973) (□), Hoffer and Forse (1990) (○).

loss depends on the initial fatness of the subject: fatter subjects will lose proportionally more fat and less lean tissue. Secondly, greater energy deficits tend towards greater losses of lean tissue. Finally, in obese subjects losses of lean tissue decrease during the first few weeks of the dieting period, but this adaptation is more effective than in their lean counterparts.

These findings should sound a note of caution to a particular group of slimmers: those who are not obese, yet who lose weight, often using VLCDs, in repeated short bouts of dieting. It is exactly this scenario in which proportionally large losses of nitrogen and lean tissue would be expected to occur. It is in this group that the perceived relationship between weight loss and fat loss is potentially harmful, since their physiological responses are geared towards the preferential preservation of their limited fat stores and proportionally greater losses of lean tissue.

It has been suggested that exercise may be beneficial during slimming by exerting a protective effect on lean tissue and thus maximizing the proportion of weight loss as fat. A recent meta-analysis has examined the results of 46 studies between 1964 and 1991 with diet only (DO) and diet plus exercise (DPE) protocols (Ballor and Poehlman, 1994). These data show that there was no significant effect of exercise on the total amount of weight lost, but the proportion of weight lost as FFM was approximately halved in both men and women. This led the authors to conclude that individuals participating in weight loss programmes should also undergo low-intensity aerobic exercise training of the order of 40–60 minute sessions of walking 5–7 days per week.

However, this analysis has been criticized because the list of studies is incomplete and in only 18 out of the 46 studies were subjects randomly assigned to DO or DPE groups (Garrow and Summerbell, 1994). But the results of individual randomized studies also suggest that the balance is in favour of a beneficial effect even if the results of the meta-analysis are slightly exaggerated.

Certainly there is no convincing evidence to suggest that exercise diminishes weight loss. This would be expected if exercise also had an appetite-stimulant effect. Nor does exercise adversely affect the composition of weight change. Exercise may therefore be encouraged in terms of its beneficial effects on other risk factors of disease, even if its effect on the metabolic response to slimming is not entirely proven (Prentice *et al.*, 1991).

The metabolic response to slimming is now well documented. The short-term physiological effects of slimming are not of such overwhelming metabolic significance as to thwart attempts to lose weight and the attainment of an appropriate body weight and composition is achievable. The challenge is now to integrate the physiological response with the behavioural and metabolic perspectives of patients to achieve a permanent and lasting resolution of their problem.

LONG-TERM CONSEQUENCES OF SLIMMING

In recent years there has been increasing interest in the question of the long-term effects of dieting, beyond the period of weight loss itself. This is particularly important for governments and health professionals concerned with long-term health at a population level.

It is well recognized that obesity is a major risk factor for many serious diseases. Obese people are two to three times more likely to die prematurely from coronary heart disease, strokes, diabetes and some forms of cancer. They have more accidents and are a greater surgical risk. Obesity also contributes to patient morbidity, with increases in hypertension, non-insulin-dependent diabetes mellitus, joint problems, depression, etc. There is a wealth of evidence to suggest that moderate weight loss can have a significant palliative effect on a wide range of obesity-related dysfunction, but the evidence that weight loss improves life expectancy is less clear.

In spite of the vast epidemiological literature on obesity, a review by Williamson and Pamuk in 1993 showed only six studies in which there was a clear beneficial effect of weight loss. Of these, some were open to methodological criticisms and the authors themselves concluded that '…the evidence from these six studies that weight loss increases longevity is equivocal'.

Since this review was written two further studies have been published on the relationship between weight loss and survival in which some of the potential errors of previous studies have been eliminated, by increasing the length of follow-up to remove any potential effects of antecedent illness. In the NHANES 1 epidemiological follow-up (Pamuk *et al.*, 1992) the relative risk of death increased with weight loss in almost all BMI and gender groups, particularly in terms of death from cardiovascular disease. Similarly, in the Harvard Alumni study (Lee and Paffenbarger, 1992), the lowest mortality was associated with weight stability. In all cases those who remained weight stable had a lower risk of death than those who either gained or lost weight. This effect was particularly marked for deaths from coronary heart disease with no significant effect on cancer deaths. Moreover, this applied whether or not the subjects were initially obese since the relative risk was similar in those with an initial BMI more or less than 25 kg m^{-2} (Figure 4.11).

This evidence is as yet inconclusive and there are a number of caveats, since collecting information on weight change in these types of study is

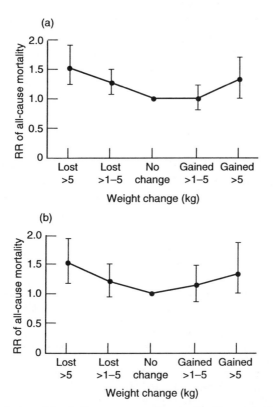

Figure 4.11 Relative risk of all-cause mortality in the Harvard Alumni Study for individuals with an initial BMI (a) less than or (b) greater than 25 kg m^{-2}. Reproduced from Lee and Paffenbarger (1992) Change in body weight and longevity. *Journal of the American Medical Association*, **268**, 2045–2049, copyright 1992 American Medical Association, with permission.

notoriously difficult. Furthermore, there is no information as to whether weight loss was consciously achieved or involuntary, the nature of any dieting regimen and the extent of any weight cycling. Experience suggests that few people who endeavour to lose weight do so at a single attempt but more usually in a number of steps interspersed with periods of weight stability or, not uncommonly, weight gain. A number of other studies have specifically examined the issue of weight cycling and are discussed elsewhere (Chapter 5).

CONCLUSIONS

It is clear that individuals with a BMI in excess of 30 kg m^{-2} have approximately twice the relative risk of death of their never obese counterparts, but it is less clear that weight loss will improve the situation. This leaves obese patients in a physiological conundrum 'dangerous to be fat: dangerous to lose it' (Prentice, 1995). In spite of this, patients will continue to want to lose weight for the foreseeable future. This is partly because, for most patients, the desire to lose weight is not motivated by the risk of death. Most are looking for quality and not quantity of life. In this respect weight loss can be extremely beneficial by improving symptoms such as glucose intolerance, hypertension, etc. Moreover, much of the desire to lose weight is not related to health issues, but rather a consequence of the current social stigmatization of obese individuals.

A deeper understanding of the metabolic response to slimming is therefore essential, but it must be concluded that measures to prevent excessive weight gain will ultimately be more successful than treatment programmes for obesity. It is worth remembering that patients do not reach a BMI of 30 without previously passing through a BMI of 25.

REFERENCES

Alban-Davies H W, McLean-Baird I, Fowler J *et al.* (1989). Metabolic responses to low- and very-low-calorie diets. *American Journal of Clinical Nutrition* **49**: 745–751.

Apfelbaum M, Bostsarron J, Lacatis D (1971). Effect of caloric restriction and excessive caloric intake on energy expenditure. *American Journal of Clinical Nutrition* **24**: 1405–1409.

Ballentyne F C, Smith J, Fleck A (1973). Albumin metabolism in fasting obese subjects. *British Journal of Nutrition* **30**: 585–593.

Ballor D L, Poehlman E T (1994). Exercise-training enhances fat free mass preservation during diet induced weight loss: a meta-analytical finding. *International Journal of Obesity* **18**: 35–40.

Barrows K and Snook J T (1987). Effect of a high-protein very-low-calorie diet on resting metabolism, thyroid hormones and energy expenditure of obese middle-aged women. *American Journal of Clinical Nutrition* **45**: 391–398.

Belko A Z, Van-Loan M, Barbieri T F, Mayclin P (1987). Diet, exercise, weight loss and energy expenditure in moderately overweight women. *International Journal of Obesity* **11**: 93–104.

Benedict F G, Miles W R, Roth P, Smith H M (1919). *Human Vitality and Efficiency Under Prolonged Restricted Diet*. Carnegie Institution of Washington, Washington DC.

Bessard T, Schutz Y, Jéquier E (1983). Energy expenditure and postprandial thermogenesis in obese women before and after weight loss. *American Journal of Clinical Nutrition* **38**: 680–693.

Bray G A (1969). The effect of caloric restriction on energy expenditure in obese patients. *Lancet* **ii**: 397–398.

Calloway D H, Spector H (1954). Nitrogen balance as related to calorie and protein intake in active young men. *American Journal of Clinical Nutrition* **2**: 405–412.

Coxon A, Kreitzman S, Brodie D, Howard A (1989). Rapid weight loss and lean tissue: evidence for comparable body composition and metabolic rate in differing rates of weight loss. *International Journal of Obesity* **13**: 179–181.

de-Boer J O, van-Es A J H, Roovers L C A et al. (1986). Adaptation of energy metabolism of overweight women to low-energy intake studied with whole-body calorimeters. *American Journal of Clinical Nutrition* **44**: 585–595.

de-Groot L C, van-Es A J, van-Raaij J M et al. (1989). Adaptation of energy metabolism of overweight women to alternating and continuous low energy intake. *American Journal of Clinical Nutrition* **50**: 1314–1323.

Diaz E, Prentice A M, Goldberg G R et al. (1992), Metabolic response to experimental overfeeding in lean and overweight healthy volunteers. *American Journal of Clinical Nutrition* **56**: 641–655.

Dore C, Wilkins D, Garrow J S (1982), Prediction of energy requirements of obese patients after massive weight loss. *Human Nutrition: Clinical Nutrition* **36C**: 41–48.

Elia M (1992). Effect of starvation and very low calorie diets on protein–energy interrelationships in lean and obese subjects. In: Schurch B, Scrimshaw N S (eds) *Protein–Energy Interactions*. IDECG, Switzerland, pp. 249–284.

Elliot D L, Goldberg L, Kuehl K S, Bennett W M (1989). Sustained depression of the resting metabolic rate after massive weight loss. *American Journal of Clinical Nutrition* **49**: 93–96.

Finer N, Swan P C, Mitchell F T (1986). Metabolic rate after massive weight loss in human obesity. *Clinical Science* **70**: 395–398.

Forbes G B (1987). Lean body mass–body fat interrelationships in humans. *Nutrition Reviews* **45**: 225–231.

Foster G D, Wadden T A, Feurer I D et al. (1990). Controlled trial of the metabolic effects of a very-low-calorie diet: short- and long-term effects. *American Journal of Clinical Nutrition* **51**: 167–172.

Fuller N J, Coward W A, Sawyer M, Elia M (1995). Total energy expenditure, basal metabolic rate and activity plus thermogenesis after vertical banded gastroplasty in obese females. *Proceedings of the Nutrition Society* (in press).

Garby L, Kurzer M S, Lammert O, Nielsen E (1988). Effect of 12 weeks' light–moderate underfeeding on 24-hour energy expenditure in normal male and female subjects. *European Journal of Clinical Nutrition* **42**: 295–300.

Garrow J, Summerbell C (1994). Meta-analysis on the effect of exercise on the composition of weight loss (letter). *International Journal of Obesity* **18**: 516–517.

Garrow J S, Webster J D (1989). Effects on weight and metabolic rate of obese women of a 3.4 MJ (800 kcal) diet. *Lancet* **i**: 1429–1431.

Goldberg G R, Black A E, Prentice A M, Coward W A (1991). No evidence of lower energy expenditure in post-obese women. *Proceedings of the Nutrition Society* **50**: 109A.

Gregory J, Foster K, Tyler H, Wiseman M (1990). *The Dietary and Nutritional Survey of British Adults*. HMSO, London.

Hainer V, Kunesova M, Stich V *et al.* (1989). Very low energy formula in the treatment of obesity. *International Journal of Obesity* **13**: 185–188.

Hendler R, Bonde A A (1988). Very-low-calorie diets with high and low protein content: impact on triiodothyronine energy expenditure and nitrogen balance. *American Journal of Clinical Nutrition* **48**: 1239–1247.

Henson L C, Poole D C, Donahoe C P, Heber D (1987). Effects of exercise training on resting energy expenditure during caloric restriction. *American Journal of Clinical Nutrition* **46**: 893–899.

Heymsfield S B, Casper K, Hearn J, Guy D (1989). Rate of weight loss during under-feeding: relation to level of physical activity. *Metabolism* **38**: 215–223.

Hill J O, Starling P B, Shields T W, Heller P A (1987). Effects of exercise and food restriction on body composition and metabolic rate in obese women. *American Journal of Clinical Nutrition* **46**: 622–630.

Hoffer L J, Forse R A (1990). Metabolic effects of a prolonged fast and hypocaloric feeding. *American Journal of Physiology* **258**: E832–E840.

Hoffer L J, Bistrian B R, Young V R *et al.* (1984). Metabolic effects of very low calorie weight reducing diets. *Journal of Clinical Investigation* **73**: 750–758.

Jansen W H (1917). Untersuchungen uber Stickstoffbilanz bei kaalorienarmer Ernahrung Deutsches. *Archiv fur klinische Medizin* **124**: 1–37.

Jebb S A, Goldberg G R, Coward W A *et al.* (1991). Effects of intermittent dieting on metabolic rate and body composition in obese women. *International Journal of Obesity* **15**: 367–374.

Keys A, Brozek J, Henschel A *et al.* (1950). *The Biology of Human Starvation*. University of Minnesota Press, Minneapolis.

Kreitzman S N, Johnson P G, Ryde S J S (1993). Dependence of weight loss during VLCD on total energy expenditure rather than on the resting metabolic rate which is associated with fat-free mass. In: Kreitzman S, Howard A (eds) *The Swansea Trial*. Smith Gordon, London, pp. 135–142.

Krotkiewski M T L, Björntorp P, Holm G (1981). The effect of a very low calorie diet with and without exercise on thyroid and sex hormones, plasma proteins, oxygen uptake, insulin and C peptide concentrations in obese women. *International Journal of Obesity* **5**: 287–293.

Landsberg L, Young J B (1983). The role of the sympathetic nervous system and catecholamines in the regulation of energy metabolism. *American Journal of Clinical Nutrition* **38**: 1018–1024.

Lee I-M, Paffenbarger R S (1992). Change in body weight and longevity. *Journal of the American Medical Association* **286**: 2045–2049.

Pamuk E R, Williamson D H, Madans J *et al.* (1992). Weight loss and mortality in a national cohort of adults 1971–1987. *American Journal of Epidemiology* **136**: 686–697.

Parkinson S A (1990). *In vivo* measurement of changes in body composition. PhD Thesis, University of Cambridge.

Pavlou K N, Krey S, Steffee W P (1989). Exercise as an adjunct to weight loss and maintenance in moderately obese subjects. *American Journal of Clinical Nutrition* **49**: 1115–1123.

Phinney S D, LaGrange B M, O'Connell M, Danforth E (1988). Effects of aerobic exercise on energy expenditure and nitrogen balance during very low calorie dieting. *Metabolism* **37**: 758–765.

Poole D C, Henson L C (1988). Effect of acute caloric restriction on work efficiency. *American Journal of Clinical Nutrition* **47**: 15–18.

Prentice A M (1988). Applications of the doubly-labelled water method in free-living adults. *Proceedings of the Nutrition Society* **47**: 259–268.

Prentice A M (1995). Is weight stability itself a reasonable goal? In: Pi Sunyer X F, Allison D B (eds) *Obesity Treatment: Establishing Goals, Improving Outcomes and Reviewing the Research Agenda.* Plenum Publishing, New York, 45–51.

Prentice A M, Goldberg G R, Jebb S A *et al.* (1991). The physiological response to slimming. *Proceedings of the Nutrition Society* **50**: 441–458.

Rabast U, Hahn A, Reiners C, Ehl M (1981). Thyroid hormone changes in obese subjects during fasting and a very-low-calorie diet. *International Journal of Obesity* **5**: 305–311.

Rattan S, Coxon A, Kreitzman S, Lemons A (1989). Maintenance of weight loss with recovery of resting metabolic rate following 8 weeks of very low calorie dieting. *International Journal of Obesity* **13**: 189–192.

Russell G F M (1987). Anorexia and bulimia nervosa penalties for fashionable slimness. In: Bender A E, Brooks L J (eds) *Body Weight Control – The Physiology, Clinical Treatment and Prevention of Obesity.* Churchill Livingstone, Edinburgh, pp. 160–169.

Ryde S J S, Saunders N H, Birks J L *et al.* (1993). The effects of VLCD on body composition. In: Kreitzman S, Howard A (eds) *The Swansea Trial.* Smith Gordon, London, pp. 31–54.

Schutz Y, Golay A, Felber J-P, Jéquier E (1984). Decreased glucose-induced thermogenesis after weight loss in obese subjects: a predisposing factor for relapse of obesity? *American Journal of Clinical Nutrition* **39**: 380–387.

van Dale D, Saris W H M, Hoor F T (1990a). Weight maintenance and resting metabolic rate 18–40 months after a diet/exercise treatment. *International Journal of Obesity* **14**: 347–359.

van Dale D, Beckers E, Schoffelen P F M *et al.* (1990b). Changes in sleeping metabolic rate and glucose induced thermogenesis during a diet or a diet/exercise treatment. *Nutrition Research* **10**: 615–626.

Webb P, Abrams T (1983). Loss of fat stores and reduction in sedentary energy expenditure from undereating. *Human Nutrition: Clinical Nutrition* **37C**: 271–282.

Webber J, Macdonald I A (1993). The relationship between changes in metabolic rate, haemodynamic variables and plasma catecholamine levels during acute starvation. *Proceedings of the Nutrition Society* **52**: 1: 53A.

Welle S L, Campbell R G (1986). Decrease in resting metabolic rate during rapid weight loss is reversed by low dose thyroid hormone treatment. *Metabolism* **35**: 289–291.

West R (1994). *Obesity.* Office of Health Economics, London.

Williamson D F, Pamuk E R (1993). The association between weight loss and increased longevity: a review of the evidence. *Annals of International Medicine* **119**(7 part 2): 731–736.

Wilson J H P, Lamberts S W J (1979). Nitrogen balances in obese patients receiving a very low calorie liquid formula diet. *American Journal of Clinical Nutrition* **32**: 612–616.

Yang M U, Barbosa-Saldivar J L, Pi-Sunyer X, Van Itallie B (1981). Metabolic effect of substituting carbohydrate for protein in a low calorie diet: a prolonged study in obese individuals. *International Obesity* **5**: 231–236.

Young V R, Haverberg L N, Bilmazes C, Munro H N (1973). Potential use of 3-methylhistidine excretion as an index of progressive reduction in muscle protein catabolism during starvation. *Metabolism* **22**: 1422– 1436.

CHAPTER 5

Health effects of weight cycling

Lauren Lissner

INTRODUCTION

In recent years, the term weight cycling has been used in the fields of nutrition and obesity to refer to repeated losses and subsequent regains of body weight in association with weight loss diets. The popular press has preferred the term 'yo-yo' dieting and has saturated the public with information and misinformation about the phenomenon. This chapter will review early studies as well as some more recent evidence relating weight cycling to health outcomes.

In the mid-1980s, a group of US-based researchers joined forces to investigate the phenomenon of weight cycling, with the following rationale. According to health surveys, weight loss dieting is very common. In one study of obese subjects, 99% of women and 90% of men reported having been on a weight loss diet (Lissner *et al.*, 1994). These figures, which describe self-reported dieting history of a sample of unsuccessful dieters seeking treatment, may over-represent the true rates of previous dieting among the obese population in general, but certainly provide evidence of a substantial failure rate. Under more controlled conditions, it has been observed that only 1% of men and 5% of women in a behavioural treatment programme showed a stable maintenance of their weight loss during a 4-year follow-up (Kramer *et al.*, 1989). This sets the stage for weight cycling. Many dieters undergo multiple cycles of weight loss and regain in pursuit of an ideal body weight.

Dieting to control body weight is not confined to overweight individuals or to adults. In one metropolitan adult population, dieting was widely reported among men and women who had never been overweight (Jeffery *et al.*, 1984). Although adherence to weight reduction diets is often assumed

Weight Control
Edited by Richard Cottrell.
Published in 1995 by Chapman & Hall, London. ISBN 0 412 73600 4

to be beneficial to health, the high rates of dieting, among the non-obese as well as the obese, have created some concern regarding potential negative health consequences.

THE METABOLIC HYPOTHESIS

Given the lack of evidence that most people who lose weight are able to sustain their losses, a 'metabolic' hypothesis was formulated. It proposed that if weight loss dieting caused permanent decreases in metabolic rate, the weight would be easily regained and every subsequent weight loss attempt would be more difficult. After an early animal study exploring this phenomenon (Brownell *et al.*, 1986), further studies of the effect of weight cycling were identified as prioritized research topics in the US (US Department of Health and Human Services, 1988).

Steen *et al.* (1988) published the first human evidence for this so-called 'metabolic hypothesis', using adolescent wrestlers as a model for weight cycling. It is a common practice among wrestlers to use restrictive diets during the wrestling season in order to place themselves in the most advantageous competing weight category. They often do this by very extreme means and display typical bulimic behaviours. The weight is then regained during the off season. In this study, two small groups of wrestlers were identified, half of whom were cyclers and the other half not. Although they were matched for age and body composition, it was found that the metabolic rates per lean body mass were lower in subjects who typically 'cut-weight' than in weight-stable wrestlers. This cross-sectional finding gave much momentum to the weight cycling endeavour, although it was not replicated prospectively (Melby *et al.*, 1990).

In a study of non-athletes (Manore *et al.*, 1991), lower relative resting energy expenditures were observed among female cyclic dieters than in non-dieters; however, unlike the study of wrestlers, the groups differed with respect to body composition. Finally, it has been shown experimentally (Jebb *et al.*, 1991; Kempen *et al.*, 1994) that the impact of weight loss on metabolic rate is fully reversible with weight regain.

WEIGHT CYCLING AND HEALTH

Although most studies did not bear out the original idea that weight cycling alters metabolic rate, the hypothesis that weight fluctuation causes chronic disease has been more difficult to prove or disprove. Early in the project, epidemiological analyses were conducted in various longitudinal databases to address this issue. It was proposed that within-individual variability in body weight might be a useful indicator of weight cycling that could be used in prospective studies to predict chronic disease. These studies are listed below and have been previously reviewed in detail (Lissner and Brownell, 1992):

- Gothenburg Prospective Study of Women (Lissner *et al.*, 1989);
- Gothenburg Prospective Study of Men (Lissner *et al.*, 1989);
- Western Electric Study (Hamm *et al.*, 1989);
- Framingham Heart Study (Lissner *et al.*, 1991);
- Baltimore Longitudinal Study of Ageing (Lissner *et al.*, 1990);
- Multiple Risk Factor Intervention Trial (MRFIT) (Blair *et al.*, 1993);
- Charleston Heart Study (Stevens and Lissner, 1990);
- Zutphen Study (Hoffmans and Kromhout, 1989).

These studies differed in their definitions of weight cycling. Some investigators used the standard deviation (or coefficient of variation) of body weight around an individual's mean or time-dependent slope, while others classified subjects as weight stable or weight cycling based on observed changes. The number of weight measurements also varied greatly between studies. The results for mortality from all causes and from cardiovascular disease are summarized separately below.

Positive associations have been observed between body weight fluctuation and all-cause mortality in most of these studies. The results are statistically significant in three of the populations described here (Lissner *et al.*, 1989, 1991; Blair *et al.*, 1993); these associations were independent of obesity and systematic weight change. Some of the studies calculated risk estimates of body weight variability relative to stability in body weight. In the Western Electric Study, the 95% confidence interval of the relative risk associated with being in the most weight-variable group ranged from 1.3 to 1.7 in men and from 1.2 to1.3 in women, the higher estimates reflecting the adjustment for mean and linear trend in BMI. In the MRFIT intervention, the increased risk associated with weight cycling, as compared with remaining weight stable, was 1.8 for a gain–loss cycle and 1.5 for a loss–gain cycle (Blair *et al.*, 1993). However, the significance of this effect was restricted primarily to men in the lowest tertile of BMI. Interestingly, a similar observation with respect to BMI was made in the Framingham women (unpublished observations).

Weight cycling and cardiovascular disease

A number of these studies examined weight fluctuation in relation to cardiovascular and coronary heart disease (reviewed by Lissner and Brownell, 1992). The majority (Hamm *et al.*, 1989; Lissner *et al.*, 1989, 1991; Blair *et al.*, 1993) observed significant, positive associations between weight fluctuation and these endpoints. Specifically, the male cohorts from Gothenburg (Lissner *et al.*, 1989) and Western Electric (Hamm *et al.*, 1989), the men and women of Framingham (Lissner *et al.*, 1991) and the men in the MRFIT trial (Blair *et al.*, 1993) all displayed elevated cardiovascular risk in association with fluctuations in body weight. In contrast, the male cohorts of Baltimore (Lissner *et al.*, 1990) and Zutphen (Stevens and Lissner, 1990) showed no association between weight fluctuation and coronary heart disease. Again, in MRFIT (Blair *et al.*, 1993) the association was only significant in the leaner group.

Weight cycling and changes in cardiovascular disease risk factors

In the Baltimore Longitudinal Study of Ageing (Lissner *et al.*, 1990), body weight variability was evaluated in relation to concomitant changes in the following dependent variables: glucose tolerance; ratio of subscapular to triceps skinfolds; ratio of waist circumference to hip circumference; systolic blood pressure; serum cholesterol; and triglyceride levels. The hypothesis here was that some of the associations that have been found between weight fluctuation and cardiovascular disease might be explained by changes in cardiovascular risk factors during weight gain that are not fully reversible with weight loss.

However, the analysis revealed that body weight variability was not significantly associated with most of these risk factors, after controlling for age, obesity and linear trend in body weight. A significant, positive association was observed between body weight variability and changes in serum glucose concentration following an oral glucose challenge, suggesting that individuals with the most variable weights had greater decreases in glucose tolerance over time. This observation of decreased glucose tolerance is consistent with two other studies of diabetes relating diabetes to weight fluctuation (Holbrook *et al.*, 1989; Blair and Paffenbarger, 1994).

The other statistically significant correlate of body weight variability in the Baltimore analysis was in the change in the ratio of subscapular to triceps skinfolds, suggesting that individuals with the most weight fluctuation had the greatest increases in truncal adiposity (Lissner *et al.*, 1990). This could be indicative of an increased centralization of body fat during the process of body weight fluctuation. However, this effect was not manifested in any changes in the waist–hip ratio. These observations may be compared with other observational studies of weight cycling in relation to centralized obesity, one of which has found positive correlations (Rodin *et al.*, 1990) and one of which found no association (Jeffery *et al.*, 1992). Furthermore, experimental studies have shown no accumulation of centralized body or visceral fat as a result of a weight loss intervention and subsequent renormalization of body weight (Jebb *et al.*, 1991; van der Kooy *et al.*, 1993). Therefore, although increased centralization of body fat with repeated weight cycles is an attractive theoretical mechanism for increased cardiovascular risks, the evidence for this is mixed at best.

INTERPRETATION OF EPIDEMIOLOGICAL
FINDINGS

The majority of available studies have shown that increased weight fluctuation is associated with subsequent occurrence of adverse health outcome (Lissner and Brownell, 1992). However, a number of methodological problems with this type of study make interpretation of these findings difficult. First, when using body weight variability as an indicator of weight cycling, different weight patterns can yield the same score. For instance, one large fluctuation may have the same score as several small fluctuations. This would be a particular problem if repeated cycles were a necessary condition for health effects. Secondly, these studies use observational data in free-living populations. In this type of study, body weight can be changing for a variety of reasons, and dieting is not usually measured. In the Gothenburg Study of Women (Lissner *et al.*, 1989), a crude indicator of dieting was available, and there was a highly significant association between having been on a diet and weight fluctuation. This suggests that some of the fluctuators were dieters. However, this crude indicator of dieting was not predictive of mortality.

In addition, the observed associations may be caused by uncontrolled confounding from a number of variables that are associated with both weight fluctuation and disease. Personality type, depression, alcohol and smoking behaviour could all result in confounding if not measured and controlled. For instance, this may be of concern in the studies showing that weight fluctuation correlates with risk of diabetes (Holbrook *et al.*, 1989; Lissner *et al.*, 1990; Blair and Paffenbarger *et al.*, 1994), a condition that is likely to be associated with weight fluctuation during its early states. In large epidemiological studies, it is difficult to identify an initially disease-free sample, and it is frequently argued that subclinical illness may be causing the weight fluctuations, rather than the reverse.

It is possible to decrease the likelihood of this explanation in two ways. In an examination of the Framingham data, a 4-year 'window' was placed between the last body weight and the first included endpoint (Lissner *et al.*, 1991). This should theoretically remove from the analysis those subjects whose weight fluctuations were occurring as a result of serious pre-existing illness. Another aspect of this problem is the possibility that many otherwise healthy individuals who go on a diet do so because they perceive themselves to be at high cardiovascular risk owing to high weight, blood pressure, cholesterol, etc. Because these individuals were at risk before they dieted, statistical adjustment for risk factors at baseline is often included in these analyses. However, this is not a fully satisfactory solution, especially since these intermediate risk factors may be part of the cardiovascular endpoint that is being examined.

PSYCHOLOGICAL FACTORS

Whether or not weight cycling is causally related to chronic disease, the psychological impact has been a cause of concern (Brownell and Rodin, 1994). Individuals with a history of weight cycling have been found to exhibit significantly more psychopathologies than weight-stable individuals of similar body weights (Foreyt *et al.*, 1995). Higher rates of eating disorders have also been suggested to be associated with repeated dieting (Polivy and Herman, 1985). Although inferences of causality in these studies require some caution, the observed associations serve as a warning that weight cycling may also carry serious psychological risks.

Another recurring theme in psychological studies of weight cycling has been the hypothesis that weight cycling causes changes in food preferences and selection patterns. Specifically, one early study showed weight-cycled animals developed a specific preference for dietary fat (Reed *et al.*, 1988), an association that theoretically could represent a causal mechanism, with respect to heart disease. More recently, two studies (Drewnowski *et al.*, 1991; Drewnowski and Holden-Wiltse, 1992) indicated an elevated preference for the sweet–fat combination among weight cyclers compared with the weight-stable obese. Although this type of association is interesting, reverse causality remains a potential problem. One might hypothesize that individuals with a strong preference for these foods would find it harder to be successful during dieting and weight maintenance.

CONCLUSIONS AND IMPLICATIONS

The majority of, but not all, prospective studies indicate that men and women undergoing body weight fluctuations are at higher risk of mortality and cardiovascular disease than individuals experiencing less fluctuation. No studies show that weight fluctuation is beneficial or that it is associated with cancer. However, the precise role of dieting remains unclear. Disease states resulting in a loss–gain or gain–loss pattern are a plausible explanation for these findings. The results presented here underscore the difficulty of using observational data to study weight cycling. More experimental data are needed; minimally, studies of subjects whose weight changes are known to be caused by dieting are critical.

On the other hand, the existing data are not consistent with the hypothesis that weight fluctuation *per se* depresses metabolic rate, so it is unlikely that dieting itself exacerbates the problem of weight gain in obese and preobese individuals. Furthermore, on the basis of existing research, there is no reason to discourage overweight patients from losing weight, even though it is likely that they will gain much of it back, for the following reason. The MRFIT and Framingham studies both suggested that any adverse effects of weight fluctuation were occurring in the relatively normal-weight subjects.

Rather than being used to deter dieting in the obese, these observations have implications for non-obese individuals, who should be advised to maintain a relatively normal weight rather than a state of fashionable underweight.

The most non-controversial message from these weight cycling studies is that overweight individuals need to be counselled in skills to maintain weight loss, and that relapse prevention should be a more central focus of weight loss programmes. Although the existing evidence relating weight cycling to adverse health outcomes must be considered equivocal, these studies have served to highlight the necessity of developing improved behavioural and nutritional strategies for maintaining weight losses and preventing weight cycling. Given the available statistics on weight regain among former dieters, it is clear that more applied research is needed in this area.

REFERENCES

Blair S N, Paffenbarger R S (1994). Influence of body weight and shape variation on incidence of cardiovascular disease, diabetes, lung disease and cancer. Presented at the 34th Annual Conference on Cardiovascular Disease Epidemiology and Prevention, March 16–19, Tampa, Florida.

Blair S N, Shaten J, Brownell K et al. (1993). Body weight change, all cause, and cause-specific mortality in the Multiple Risk Factor Intervention Trial. *Annals of Internal Medicine* 119: 749–757.

Brownell K D, Rodin J (1994). Medical, metabolic and psychological effects of weight cycling. *Archives of Internal Medicine* 154: 1325–1330.

Brownell K, Greenwood M R C, Stellan E, Shrager E E (1986). The effects of repeated cycles of weight loss and regain in rats. *Physiology and Behaviour* 38: 459–464.

Drewnowski A, Holden-Wiltse J (1992). Taste responses and food preferences in obese women: effects of weight cycling. *International Journal of Obesity* 16: 639–648.

Drewnowski A, Kurth C, Rahaim J E (1991). Taste preferences in human obesity: environmental and familial factors. *American Journal of Clinical Nutrition* 54: 635–641.

Foreyt J B, Brunner R L, St Jeor S T, Goodrick G K (1995). Psychological correlates of weight fluctuation. *International Journal of Eating Disorders* (in press).

Hamm P B, Shekelle R B, Stamler J (1989). Large fluctuations in body weight during young adulthood and 25-year risk of coronary death in men. *American Journal of Epidemiology* 129: 312–318.

Hoffmans M D A F, Kromhout D (1989). Changes in BMI in relation to myocardial infarction incidence and mortality (abstract 25). *International Journal of Obesity* 13 (Suppl. 1).

Holbrook T L, Barret-Connor E, Wingard D L (1989). The association of lifetime weight and weight control patterns with diabetes among men and women in an adult community. *International Journal of Obesity* 13: 723–729.

Jebb S A, Goldberg G R, Coward W A et al. (1991). Effects of weight cycling caused by intermittent dieting on metabolic rate and body composition in obese women. *International Journal of Obesity* 15: 367–374.

Jeffery R W, Folsom A R, Luepker R V *et al.* (1984). Prevalence of overweight and weight loss behaviour in a metropolitan adult population: The Minnesota Heart Survey Experience. *American Journal of Public Health* **74**: 349–352.

Jeffery R W, Wing R R, French S A (1992). Weight cycling and cardiovascular risk factors in obese men and women. *American Journal of Clinical Nutrition* **55**: 641–644.

Kempen K P G, Saris W H M, van Baak M A (1994). A 1-year weight cycle has no effect on body composition and energy expenditure in obese females (abstract). *International Journal of Obesity* **18**: 52.

Kramer F M, Jeffrey R W, Forster J L, Snell M K (1989). Long-term follow-up of behavioural treatment for obesity: patterns of weight regain among men and women. *International Journal of Obesity* **13**: 123–136.

Lissner L, Brownell K (1992). Weight cycling, mortality and cardiovascular disease: a review of epidemiological findings. In: Björntorp P, Brodoff B (eds) *Obesity*. J B Lippincott, Philadelphia, pp. 653–661.

Lissner L, Bengtsson C, Lapidus L *et al.* (1989). Body weight variability and mortality in the Gothenburg Prospective Studies of Men and Women. In: Björntorp P, Rössner S (eds) *Obesity in Europe 88*. Libbey, London, pp. 55–60.

Lissner L, Andrew R, Muller D, Shimokata H (1990). Body weight variability in men: metabolic rate, health and longevity. *International Journal of Obesity* **14**: 373–383.

Lissner L, Odell P, D'Agostino R *et al.* (1991). Variability of body weight and health outcomes in the Framingham population. *New England Journal of Medicine* **324**: 1839–1844.

Lissner L, Bengtsson C, Bouchard C *et al.* (1994). The natural history of obesity in an obese population and associations with selected cardiovascular risk factors. *International Journal of Obesity* **18**: 441–447.

Manore M M, Berty T E, Skinner J S, Carrol S S (1991). Energy expenditure at rest and during exercise in non-obese female cyclic dieters and in non-dieting control subjects. *American Journal of Clinical Nutrition* **54**: 41–46.

Melby C L, Schmidt D, Corrigan D (1990). Resting metabolic rate in weight-cycling collegiate wrestlers compared with physically active, non-cycling control subjects. *American Journal of Clinical Nutrition* **52**: 409–414.

Polivy J, Herman C P (1985). Dieting and bingeing: a causal analysis. *American Journal of Psychology* **40**: 193–201.

Reed D R, Contrereas R J, Maggio C *et al.* (1988). Weight cycling in female rats increases dietary fat selection and adiposity. *Physiology and Behaviour* **42**: 389–395.

Rodin J, Radke-Sharpe N, Rebuffé-Scrive M, Greenwood M R C (1990). Weight cycling and fat distribution. *International Journal of Obesity* **14**: 303–310.

Steen S N, Oppiger R A, Brownell K D (1988). Metabolic effects of repeated weight loss and regain in adolescent wrestlers. *JAMA* **260**: 47–50.

Stevens J, Lissner L (1990). Body weight variability and mortality in the Charleston Heart Study. *International Journal of Obesity* **14**: 385–386.

US Department of Health and Human Services (1988). *The Surgeon General's Report on Nutrition and Health*, Publication No. 88–50210. Government Printing Office, Washington DC.

van der Kooy K, Leenen R, Seidell J *et al.* (1993). Effect of weight cycle on visceral fat accumulation. *American Journal of Clinical Nutrition* **58**: 853–857.

CHAPTER 6

Food preferences and body weight control

France Bellisle

INTRODUCTION

There is an abundant scientific literature describing research into the behavioural causes of human obesity. However, the numerous hypotheses put forward over the years have led to very few convincing conclusions. In 1981, Spitzer and Rodin published a review of psychophysiological and behavioural studies comparing obese subjects with a control group of normal weight. They concluded that no characteristic could be regarded as being specific to obese persons. Most of the studies quoted did not establish any difference between obese persons and the control group, be it in the daily energy intake, eating habits or behaviour observed in the laboratory. The studies that reported differences between obese persons and the control group were contradictory. The conclusion must be that there is a great diversity of behaviour among obese populations just as there is among people of normal weight. This extreme intra-group diversity makes it difficult, or even impossible, to establish statistically (and scientifically) significant inter-group differences.

FOOD PREFERENCES AND OBESITY

However, some more recent work points to differences in food preferences between obese persons and control groups of normal weight. Enns *et al.* (1979) had their subjects taste sugared solutions and observed among both children and adults that corporal adiposity was inversely correlated to a preference for sugar. In contrast, Warwick and Schiffman (1990) reported that, in food stimuli consisting of fat and sugar, obese youngsters preferred

Weight Control
Edited by Richard Cottrell.
Published in 1995 by Chapman & Hall, London. ISBN 0 412 73600 4

a mixture of 17% fat and 12.4% sucrose, while subjects of normal weight enjoyed more fat: 24.6% fat and 11.3% sucrose.

The extensive work carried out by Drewnowski supports the thesis of a marked fondness for fats among obese persons (accompanied by less of a liking for sugar) than among persons of normal weight. These studies, based on sensory evaluation, often used foodstuffs (ice cream, for example) as stimuli rather than aqueous solutions. The volunteers briefly tasted samples of these foods and spat them out. They then gave the sample various marks representing their perception of the product. When 20 different mixtures of milk, cream and sugar (Drewnowski *et al.*, 1985) were assessed in this way, obese persons preferred very fatty stimuli (at least 34% fat) with little sugar (less than 5% sucrose) compared with the control group (20% fat, 10% sucrose). After slimming, formerly obese persons showed a partiality for strong concentrations of fat and sugar. Drewnowski and Holden-Wiltse (1992) have also demonstrated that the 'yo-yo syndrome' is the cause of changes in food preferences. While preferences for sugared solutions seemed to be the same among obese persons with a stable body weight and obese persons with a very unstable body weight, the latter showed a more marked liking for ice creams and sweet desserts. This observation suggests that large weight fluctuations in obese persons can be linked to an increased liking for foods that are both sweet and rich in fat.

Preferences for fat-rich foods among obese Americans are confirmed by studies based on different methodologies. For instance, Drewnowski *et al.* (1992) demonstrated that when volunteers drew up a list of their 10 favourite foods, obese persons most often chose fatty foods. Drewnowski (1988) observes, on the basis of the results of the National Health and Nutrition Examinations Surveys (1976–1980), that many of the favourite foods of Americans are sweet and/or rich in fats. Furthermore, sugar is not the main source of energy in many popular sweet foods: chocolate, cake, ice cream, milk drinks, etc. In effect, these products derive most of their calories from the fat that they contain.

It is important to check the observations made during sensory tests in the laboratory by consumption studies. In fact, it is not certain that preferences expressed in the artificial circumstances of tests, when food is not swallowed, are actually representative of food choices in daily life (Pangborn and Giovanni, 1984; Lucas and Bellisle, 1987). Theoretical considerations (Geiselman and Novin, 1982; Fullerton *et al.* 1985) suggest that carbohydrates, and sugars in particular, might play a role in bulimia (bulimia nervosa) and obesity (because of the secretion of β-endorphins following the consumption of sugar). Studies through surveys, on the other hand, reveal that there is no link between obesity and the consumption of carbohydrates. Garn *et al.* (1980), after interviewing 4970 American adolescents, report no observation that could indicate more marked preferences among obese persons for sweet foods. Lewis *et al.* (1992) studied the consumption of 4000 foodstuffs among 30 770 Americans of all ages and noted that excess body weight is not linked to the consumption of added sugar.

FAT INTAKE AND FAT PREFERENCE IN THE GENESIS OF OBESITY

Many recent studies emphasize that the ingestion of fat can favour the development and maintenance of obesity. While a high consumption of carbohydrates gives rise to an increased oxidation of carbohydrates, excessive consumption of fats does not give rise to the oxidation of fats and the surplus fats are therefore stored in the organism's reserves (Verboeket-van de Venne *et al.*, 1994). This mechanism is certainly responsible for the excess body fat reserves in people who, in developed societies, obtain over 40% of their daily energy intake from fats, despite repeated recommendations from nutritionists. An excessive intake of fats could be favoured by the low satiating power of lipids (Blundell and Burley, 1990) and by their high energy density (9 kcal g^{-1}, as opposed to 4 kcal g^{-1} for proteins and carbohydrates). Warwick and Schiffman (1992) showed that the pleasant orosensory qualities of lipids stimulate consumption, whereas their post-absorptive metabolism facilitates the depositing and accumulation of body fats.

Many new findings cumulatively reinforce the determining role of the intake of lipids in the occurrence of obesity. Yet while certain surveys show that obese persons consume more fats than nutritional recommendations (Creff and Herscberg, 1979), it has still not been convincingly demonstrated that obese persons consume more fat than persons of normal weight. It is as if, in a given population with a given diet, some individuals are more susceptible to obesity than the majority of their peers, while eating just like everyone else. This hypothesis of a greater susceptibility among certain people is reinforced by some very recent work demonstrating a very strong genetic element in obesity (Bouchard, 1994).

GENETIC PREDISPOSITION

While the genes predisposing to obesity are distributed throughout the human species, background, environment and society can play a part in encouraging the development of obesity. It has been demonstrated many times that in developed societies there is no correlation between individual energy intake and body weight (Rolland-Cachera *et al.*, 1986, 1988, 1990); however, there is a larger proportion of obese persons in certain strata of the population, in certain socioeconomic groups that are characterized by higher energy intakes. For instance, it has been demonstrated that among French children and adults the proportion of heavy or obese individuals is higher in those socio-professional categories in which daily energy intakes are the highest. In workers' families, the proportion of obese children is higher than in the families of executives. And the energy intake is higher among the working class population.

However, obese children from a particular background do not eat more than (or differently from) their slim friends. A characteristic energy intake in a given milieu challenges individual adaptation capacities largely determined by the genetic heritage. The higher the intake, the greater the number of individuals incapable of regulating their energy reserves and maintaining a normal weight. The more a society eats, the greater the prevalence of obesity, whereas obese persons do not necessarily eat more than the others.

These comparisons between groups of people exposed to a different risk, determined by the physical or social environment, are more revealing here than case–control group comparisons (between obese persons and persons of normal weight). Comparisons between populations are sources of hypotheses as to the behaviour patterns involved in the aetiology of obesity. These hypotheses must then be tested in the laboratory or in the field.

REFERENCES

Blundell J E, Burley V J (1990). Evaluation of the satiating power of dietary fat in man. In: Oomura Y *et al.* (eds) *Progress in Obesity Research*. John Libbey, London, pp. 453–457.

Bouchard C (1994). *Génétique et Obésité*. Ardix Médical, Paris.

Creff A F, Herscberg A D (1979). *Obésité*. Masson, Paris.

Drewnowski A (1988). Sweet foods and sweeteners in the US diet. In: Bray G A *et al.* (eds) *Diet and Obesity*. Japan Sci Soc Press, Tokyo, pp. 153–161.

Drewnowski A, Holden-Wiltse J (1992). Taste responses and food preference in obese women: effects of weight cycling. *International Journal of Obesity* **16**: 639–648.

Drewnowski A, Brunzell J D, Sande K *et al.* (1985). Sweet tooth reconsidered: taste responsiveness in human obesity. *Physiology and Behaviour* **35**: 617–622.

Drewnowski A, Kurth C, Holden-Wiltse, Saari J (1992). Food preferences in human obesity: carbohydrates versus fats. *Appetite* **18**: 207–221.

Enns M P, Van Itallie T B, Grinker J A (1979). Contributions of age, sex and degree of fatness on preferences and magnitude estimations for sucrose in humans. *Physiology and Behaviour* **22**: 999–1003.

Fullerton D T, Getto C J, Swift W J, Carlson I H (1985). Sugar, opioids and binge eating. *Brain Research Bulletin* **14**: 673–680.

Garn S M, Solomon M A, Cole P E (1980). Sugar-food intake of obese and lean adolescents. *Ecology of Food and Nutrition* **9**: 219–222.

Geiselman P J, Novin D (1982). The role of carbohydrates in appetite, hunger and obesity. *Appetite* **3**: 203–223.

Lewis C J, Park Y K, Dexter P B, Yetley E A (1992) Nutrient intakes and body weights of persons consuming high and moderate levels of added sugars. *Journal of the American Dietetic Association* **92**: 708–713.

Lucas F, Bellisle F (1987). The measurement of food preferences in humans: do taste-and-spit tests predict consumption? *Physiology and Behaviour* **39**: 739–743.

Pangborn R M, Giovanni M E (1984). Dietary intake of sweet foods and of dairy fats and resultant gustatory responses to sugar in lemonade and to fat in milk. *Appetite* **5**: 317–327.

Rolland-Cachera M F, Bellisle F (1986). No correlation between adiposity and food intake: why are working class children fatter? *American Journal of Clinical Nutrition* **44**: 779–787.

Rolland-Cahera M F, Deheeger M, Péquignot F *et al.* (1988). Adiposity and food intake in young children: the environmental challenge to individual susceptibility. *British Medical Journal* **296**: 1037–1038.

Rolland-Cachera M F, Bellisle F, Tichet J *et al.* (1990). Relationship between adiposity and food intake: an example of pseudo-contradictory results obtained in case-control versus between-population studies. *International Journal of Epidemiology* **19**: 571–577.

Spitzer L, Rodin J (1981). Human eating behaviour: a critical review of studies in normal weight and overweight individuals. *Appetite* **2**: 293329.

Verboeket-van de Venne W P H G, Westerterp K R, ten Hoor F (1994). Substrate utilization in man: effects of dietary fat and carbohydrate. *Metabolism* **43**: 152–156.

Warwick Z S, Schiffman S S (1990). Sensory evaluations of fat:sucrose and fat:salt mixtures: relationship to age and weight status. *Physiology and Behaviour* **48**: 633–636.

Warwick Z S, Schiffman S S (1992). Role of dietary fat in calorie intake and weight gain. *Neuroscience and Biobehavioural Review* **16**: 585–596.

CHAPTER 7

Psychological aspects of obesity

Volker Pudel

INTRODUCTION

From a psychological point of view, the aetiology of obesity is not as clear as it used to be 40 years ago. Any historical review of the development of the basic ideas on the psychology of obesity leads, today, to more questions than answers. As well as the many publications of Hilde Bruch (e.g. Bruch, 1973), who dealt primarily with the 'fat child', the works of Ferster, Nurnberger, and Levitt (e.g. Ferster *et al.*, 1962) are foundation documents concerning behavioural research. At that time, a concept called 'control of eating' was introduced. This included a substantial section on possible obesity therapy and was the basic influence on concepts for two or three decades. Brillat-Savarin (1971) paraphrased this as 'moderation while eating, restraint while sleeping and making an effort while walking or riding'. These ideas led to a campaign in the media saying 'eating and keeping fit are both important factors', while Wallis (1975) explained that 'adipose people eat too much and don't exercise enough, or they might eat normally and don't do any exercise or perhaps they eat far too much and do regular exercise'.

EARLY PSYCHOLOGICAL THEORIES

This simple principle of an energy balance affected psychological research in two ways.

1. In several studies, many different tests were used to characterize the personality of adipose people. These studies were based on the hypothesis

Weight Control
Edited by Richard Cottrell.
Published in 1995 by Chapman & Hall, London. ISBN 0 412 73600 4

that certain neurotic characteristics would explain the excessive ingestion by obese people as an 'oral compensation mechanism'. If correct, evidence in support of this hypothesis would lead to the development of new concepts in the psychotherapy of the patient (Pudel, 1982). However, almost all studies failed to show a relevant difference between 'normal' and obese persons. It was established that there were no typical features of personality that were characteristic of all obese people (Pudel and Westenhöfer, 1991).

2. The second initial stage of behavioural research used experimental studies, in which the eating habits of test subjects under controlled conditions were directly observed. This approach was also based on the hypothesis that fat people eat more than normal subjects. It was considered important to define and study the different conditions that are responsible for this excessive eating. A substantial number of creative experiments were published. The first of these, Schachter's (1968) classic study leading to the 'externality theory', merits particular mention. According to this theory, there are external stimuli influencing the eating habits of obese people, which means that their appetite and their feeling of repletion are not just controlled by 'internal, biological signals', but rely on environmental signals such as the sight of food or an appetizing preparation. Further experiments showed that the obese persons more often exhibited hyperphagia under stress. In addition, it was found that their process of repletion slowed down. Through this and similar experimental results in the 1970s an almost complete picture of the eating behaviour of obese people took shape. This seemed to explain why 'fat people' eat so. Underlying this were the hypothetical eating pattern disturbances that were seen to result from inadequate learning processes (Schacter, 1971).

The state of excess food availability in the industrialized nations has created the conditions that allow an above average manifestation of these interferences in food consumption. This led to a further understanding of the behavioural theory of intervention. The adipose patient has to learn a new way of eating, and has to adjust to an undisturbed eating behaviour in order to keep weight normal after having finished a reduction diet. Today, this basic therapy of a combination of diet and behaviour is still used, although the earlier hypotheses and theories have now been modified. That this innovative behaviour therapy was based on an insufficient view of obesity was already noted by Stunkard (1975) when he established that the expected success of an obesity treatment did not always occur after the introduction of behaviour therapy.

It is still a problem to attain a long-term stabilization of weight that has been reduced through a diet, although it should be noted that better results are achieved than by using separate dietary measures (Perri *et al.*, 1984).

EMERGENCE OF THE RESTRAINED EATER

That same year, 1975, two studies were conducted based on a different supposition, in which a certain category of persons were described as 'restrained eaters' (Herman and Polivy, 1975). We have called them 'latent obese persons' (Pudel *et al.*, 1975). What these people have in common is that they are more or less normal weight but their eating behaviour shows a similarity to obese people. The concept of 'restrained eating' is internationally accepted to characterize an eating behaviour in which cognitive control is the most important factor. Restrained eaters' count calories, do not finish meals to the point of satisfying hunger, choose low-calorie food, avoid sweets and fat and permanently look after their weight and eating behaviour; or they go on an intermittent diet. Test methods introduced by Herman and Polivy (1984) and Stunkard and Messick (1985) identify 'restrained eaters' or determine 'the amount of cognitive control during meals'. After this concept had been accepted and was used in various experiments, the knowledge gained led to a better understanding of obesity.

RESTRAINED EATING AND OBESITY

The extent to which subjects cognitively control their own eating behaviour has a greater influence on this behaviour, and its susceptibility to problems, than the body weight. This effect is the same whether subjects are of normal weight or overweight, therefore people who are within a normal weight range as well as those who are overweight can be restricted eaters or impulsive eaters. Behaviour that was held to be typical of obese people in fact directly relates to restricted eaters, independent of their weight. Because of this observation, the hypothesis of a disturbed eating behaviour characteristic of obese people was abandoned. Countless studies in the following years confirmed that there are no differences in eating patterns related to body weight, if the cognitive control of eating behaviour by the experimental subjects is taken into account. These studies laid the foundation for the hypothesis that obesity cannot be taken as a diagnostic category in the Diagnostic and Statistical Manual of Mental Disorders, 'because it does not conform to marked psychological behavioural symptoms in general' (Koehler and Saß, 1984).

One may ask how this 'research error' could occur, especially since the experiments of the 1960s and early 1970s defined concepts of therapy still in use. A possible explanation may be that obese people who volunteered themselves for scientific study were not only obese, but also restricted eaters. It is not difficult to envisage that overweight people who always cognitively control their eating behaviour are more highly motivated to take part in clinical or experimental studies, because they hope for new knowledge or professional help. Through this self-selection the variables of overweight and 'restraint' were confused and the typical characteristics attributed to obese people were, in fact, not specific to them but were rather typical of 'restricted eaters'. Thus, for example, a notice in a newspaper for a dietary study would attract a response from a preponderance of 'restricted eaters', whereas a notice for pudding taste tests would appeal more to the 'unrestricted eater'. Puddings, associated with becoming fat, increase fears of weight gain for restricted eaters.

BULIMIA NERVOSA

Behavioural research into obesity unexpectedly received a new boost from a totally different direction. In 1979, the clinical condition of bulimia nervosa was described by Russell (1979). Characteristic of this eating disorder is an extreme fear of weight gain or an intense desire to lose weight. This results in extreme diets, a highly restrictive eating pattern, the selection of 'slimming products' as well as the avoidance of all high-calorie foods. The more rigidly this principle is implemented, the more often these people (in the last few years mostly young women, although an increasing number of men) experience intense hunger attacks. These can occur several times a day. In order to master the fear of weight gain, patients resort to self-induced vomiting or the use of laxatives or diuretics. A diagnosis of the disease bulimia nervosa eventually becomes apparent. The hunger attacks become more frequent and increase in intensity, but in almost all cases the disease begins with a strict 'slimming diet'. The epidemic appearance of bulimia in Germany began in the mid-1960s and now has an estimated prevalence of approximately 2.5–4% of the total German population over 14 years of age (Deutsche Gesellschaft für Ernährung, 1992).

The 1960s were symbolized by a change in the ideals of beauty. This is expressed in the publicity surrounding 'Twiggy' at the time, the decreasing weight of models in the men's magazine *Playboy*, the propagation of new and supposedly more effective crash diets as well as the adoption of an 'ideal' body weight that corresponded to a BMI of barely 20. The message that had to be grasped by every citizen was plain and simple: 'Body weight depends on eating patterns. It can be easily raised or lowered, as one wishes.' The weight of a person was thus presented as a function of cognitive efforts. The treatment of overweight people also changed to a cognitive behaviour therapy with countless rules and exercises, calorie counting and nutrient awareness.

Many scientists interested in obesity turned their attention to bulimia. Obviously, parallels had to be drawn between the two. The long-term restrictive eating patterns followed by bulimic patients as a result of intensive self-motivation were the aim of obesity therapy, although obese patients do not usually exhibit such high compliance. In addition, it was not difficult to transfer the concept of 'restricted eating' to bulimic behaviour.

Soon tests showed that bulimic patients have an extremely restricted eating pattern that is characterized by a high susceptibility.

Suddenly studies and results that had been published years before, but not brought to light, were newly 'discovered'. The pattern of fat distribution and its specific risks that Vague had already described in 1947 is an example of this (Hauner, 1987), as is the Minnesota Study of Keys *et al.* (1950). Thirty-six young, healthy men who avoided their US military duty in 1944 were supplied with only 50% of their usual nourishment in this 'starvation study'. They not only lost 25% of their starting weight, but also reacted with many symptoms that are known to bulimia sufferers and dieters: permanent thoughts of food, hunger attacks, lack of satisfaction even after large meals, reduction of psychological well-being and achievement capabilities, depressive moods and sexual dysfunction to name but a few. A reduction in the basic metabolic rate of 40% was recorded by indirect calorimetry. In the following 3 months' rehabilitation it was established that, when the starting weight was regained, the fat mass had increased, and that, in turn, influenced the free fats. It should be pointed out that the experimental conditions in the Minnesota Study, that is the reduction of food intake to 50%, correspond to the most widely adopted method of weight loss used in Germany. Out of those who had, up to 1980, already carried out a reduction diet, 55% reported that they 'had only eaten half'.

STRICT CONTROL AND THE DISTURBANCE OF EATING BEHAVIOUR

In a representative survey in Germany it was established that approximately 50% of all women and 25% of all men had already taken part in a reduction diet. It was further asked, from the subjective point of view of the interviewees, if eating patterns were connected with difficulties or were unproblematic. The report shows that, in a wide population sample, women as well as men reported symptoms that exist as extreme examples in eating-disturbed patients (Westenhöfer and Pudel, 1990). This is also already documented in the study of Keys *et al.* (1950). If the frequency of diets and problems in eating behaviour are observed together, it can be seen that over 90% of those who implemented more than three diets reported eating problems, while only 27% of those who had not been on a diet reported difficulties. This correlative relationship, when taken with the observations of Keys and others, supports the hypothesis that a strict calorie restriction, in whatever form, can lead to an increased disturbance of eating behaviour.

A test 'questionnaire about the eating behaviour' [original version by Stunkard and Messick (1985), German version by Pudel and Westenhöfer (1989)] examined, among other things, the extent of cognitive control of eating behaviour and its disturbance in individual cases. An examination of 44 800 participants in a weight reduction programme, the Four Seasons Programme, yielded a very clear result. A highly significant, three-dimensional correlation between relative weight (based on BMI), cognitive control and the presence of eating disturbance exists. High disturbance, when combined with poor cognitive control, results in the highest BMI. High control but low disturbance on its own leads to a low BMI. The higher the disturbance and the lower the cognitive control that can be demonstrated in the test, the more the weight of the participants increases. The success rate in a weight reduction programme involving 12 months of training provided consistent evidence: participants with low disturbance and high control were successful in almost 60% of cases, while only 30% of participants with high disturbance and low control were successful (Westenhöfer, 1991a).

There is no obvious need to explain or discuss the meaning of cognitive control further, but the category 'proneness to malfunction of eating behaviour' presents greater problems. While it is true that the description of these eating disorders is straightforward (since the symptoms voracious appetite, craving for sweets, stress eating, unsatisfiable hunger, etc. have been known for some time), the genesis of the proneness to malfunction of eating behaviour remained unclear. The seemingly obvious hypothesis that adopting a restrictive diet, or reducing weight, increases the proneness to malfunction cannot be confirmed by correlations alone.

COUNTER-REGULATION

Herman and Polivy (1984) have contributed additional information to the problem with a significant experiment. Restrained and unrestrained eaters participated in a taste test in which they tried different sorts of ice cream. It was expected that the restrained eaters would more strictly control themselves than the unrestrained eaters, and would consume less of the ice cream. In fact, the experiments led to the opposite result. Restrained eaters consumed significantly more ice cream than unrestrained eaters, but only when given one or two milkshakes before the experiment began. If denied the welcome milkshake, the participants behaved as predicted according to their classification: the restrained eaters ate less and the unrestrained eaters ate more. Different variations of the experiment prove that the interpretation given by the authors is correct. If the same milkshake is offered as a low-calorie 'light drink', then the restrained eaters eat little, as expected; on the other hand, they take more ice cream when the milkshake is labelled 'calorie bomb'.

This experiment illustrates a phenomenon that for some time has been known as 'counter-regulation'. The milkshake given before the experiment exceeds a cognitive calorie intake limit that the restrained eater has defined. The daily limit is now surpassed and the restrained thinks 'it no longer matters how much ice cream I eat'. The principle of self-imposed cognitive control works only as long as it is not violated. If it is subjectively breached, the whole system of self-control collapses, although a few milkshakes more or less should not initiate the breakdown. Thus, the term 'counter-regulation' describes the condition in which an incident that is, in itself, negligible leads to the collapse of the whole control system. A strict cognitive control of one's eating behaviour will only be permanently effective if no counter-regulation occurs. Therefore, the sudden hunger attacks suffered by bulimic patients are nothing more than counter-regulations that block any control. Or, to put it another way, the disturbance of eating behaviour illustrates the failure of cognitive control. In this way, the entry into the state of counter-regulation is an essential factor in the proneness to malfunction.

INDIVIDUAL VARIABILITY

Westenhöfer (1991b) drew attention to an inconsistency in this theoretical description of the condition. 'One problem in drawing a causal connection between restrained eating and sudden eating attacks', he wrote, 'can be seen in the fact that restrained eating behaviour is not a uniform category, that the group of restrained eaters is not an homogenous group, and that not all of the restrained eaters suffer eating attacks or a disturbance of eating behaviour at all'.

In various empirical surveys, sometimes with very large groups, for example about 50 000 participants in a weight-reducing programme, Westenhöfer discovered that the category 'restrained eating' is certainly not uniform. He explained (and developed additional precise tests for the 'questionnaire about eating behaviour') that there are different ways to curb one's eating behaviour, but he considers that it comes down to two basic strategies that either increase or reduce the possibility of eating disorders. He makes a distinction between rigid control strategies and flexible control. Rigid control is based on firm, strictly defined intentions of behaviour, which often are absolute. Phrases such as 'I will never again...', 'I will always...', 'I will from now on...' are typical rigid strategies that follow the all-or-nothing principle. Rigid control will always be put out of order by counter-regulation because harmless incidents breach the strictly drawn borderlines. Flexible control aims at more general and lasting attitudes and behaviour patterns, and allows for a possible correction of behaviour at any point in time. It is a sort of self-control that leaves either little or no room for counter-regulation. Slight divergencies, caused by negligible incidents, are not regarded as a violation of one's self-defined limits, but leave room for corrections. Instead of taking an attitude such as 'No more sweets from now on', which is apt to cause counter-regulation after consuming just a single piece of chocolate, one is better off saying 'Next week, I will try to get by with only one chocolate bar'.

Westenhöfer (1991b) found empirical evidence that rigid control increases the possibility of malfunction, whereas flexible control promotes a more undisturbed eating behaviour. All of the training programmes for obese patients that are based on cognitive approaches concentrate on the practice of cognitive control. Rigid strategies ought to be removed from those programmes that still offer a mixture of rigid and flexible control mechanisms, since they tend to contribute to eating disorders – despite their original intention. Thus, the problems of cognitive control demonstrated by behavioural studies will be resolved, at least to some extent, if the results of this research are applied in practical obesity therapy.

DIETARY MACRONUTRIENT SELECTION AND BODY WEIGHT CONTROL

The following questions still remain unanswered: 'Do people who are suffering from obesity really have a higher or lower intake of food energy than people with a normal weight' and 'Do obese people take in food energy above average during the dynamic phase of weight increase?'. Almost all of the studies that have compared self-reported nutrition records kept by normal and overweight persons show no relevant differences in caloric intake (Pudel and Westenhöfer, 1991). Energy intake studies from 200 000 people are almost congruent – in spite of the different weights of the participants. On the other hand, direct and indirect measurements of energy utilization (for example using calorimetry or doubly labelled water) do not indicate that obese people, on average, have a generally low resting metabolic rate, although this is the case with some individuals. These cases are not as common, though, as obese patients think, and therefore a low resting metabolism is not the main cause of the eating disorders of the majority. However, analyses that go beyond mere calorie intake suggest that, in the case of obesity, the relative intake of fat is increased whereas the supply of carbohydrates is reduced.

Unlike carbohydrates, fat intake is probably of greater importance to weight regulation than has been assumed to date, because fat intake is not regulated in an exact, i.e. in an energy-equivalent, way. Subjects who reduced their fat intake for more that 12 months were twice as successful in reaching their target weight than those participants who lost weight solely by reducing carbohydrates (Pudel and Westenhöfer, 1992).

In other studies (Kendall *et al.*, 1991; Schlundt *et al.*, 1993) as well as in my own research, a significantly higher loss of weight could be observed – in spite of an *ad libitum* diet – in a group of people who were given a diet with a reduced fat content. In the study by Kendall *et al.* (1991), in which some test subjects were nourished *ad libitum* with a low-fat diet and others with a normal-fat diet for 11 weeks on two occasions, a precise regulation of food intake was observed at an average of 1.4 kg per day. When the intake of fat was reduced but the volume taken in remained unchanged, the result was a significantly greater loss of weight. One point of criticism of all of these studies is that the control group, despite a larger dietary fat supply, also lost weight, but not to the same extent as the low-fat group. It needs to be mentioned that comparable studies, in which the fat content was uninfluenced but the carbohydrate content was varied by providing one group with food sweetened with sucrose or artificial sweeteners, did not result in differences in weight reduction.

From a psychological point of view, two more aspects need to be mentioned in regard to attitudes that have been propagated to obese patients for decades (Foreyt, 1977; Perri *et al.*, 1984; Brownell and Wadden, 1986). It has been uncontested for some years that there is a genetic predisposition in weight regulation and in energy metabolism (Bouchard and Tremblay, 1990; Bouchard *et al.*, 1990), although it is unclear what implications either for therapy or for prevention follow from this fact. For some years it seems to have been increasingly accepted that humans, unlike other species, under normal conditions do not use carbohydrates for *de novo* lipid biosynthesis, although this metabolic pathway is available at a daily carbohydrate intake above 500 g. But consumption of such a large amount of carbohydrate is unlikely, at least if it is provided as food containing complex carbohydrates. These studies seem to supply a plausible explanation for the research mentioned above that showed greater loss of weight, in spite of an *ad libitum* diet, when the fat content of the diet was reduced. This can be regarded as an important insight into the prevention and therapy of obesity as far as the diet is concerned.

SUCCESSFUL AND UNSUCCESSFUL WEIGHT CONTROL STRATEGIES

A critical evaluation of the history of obesity research since the time when obesity began its epidemic spread in affluent societies demonstrates which strategies are nonsensical and do not tend to be successful. One of those strategies is the overall caloric mathematics that deals with fat and carbohydrates as having equal value. This approach must also be regarded as a rigid control strategy. Secondly, the statement that everybody could reach a desired weight, and to do so is merely a question of nutrition, and therefore indirectly a question of controlled eating behaviour, is inadequate. This unidimensional approach is complicated by the fact that the principle of energy balance is still valid, but in a restricted way. One only loses weight when one has a negative energy balance between nutrient intake and exercise. However, obesity therapy is not only the initial loss of weight, but also the maintenance of a reduced weight. Clinical studies show that with formula diets it is possible even for very obese patients to reduce weight in a relatively short period of time without major subjective problems. But still, in many cases, weight increases again – in spite of behaviour therapy. This weight increase represents failure for patients and therapists. But why is weight gain unavoidable?

Is it possible that the maintenance of a reduced weight is a continuous battle against biological mechanisms that can only be won by the lifetime task of hunger management? Or does weight management fail in one's mind in the presence of food abundance, because freedom of choice and availability of food influence human behaviour so strongly that behaviour patterns developed in times of need produce failure?

These questions remain unanswered, but they need to be considered, not least because of the millions of overweight people in whom body weight is seen by physicians as an indicator of health and by society as a measure of self-esteem and happiness. There are not many formerly overweight people, but there are plenty of previously overweight people who are still overweight and have all the psychological attributes that are specific for people who are used to failure. It appears that the ineffectiveness of obesity therapy cannot be explained by 'non-compliance' alone.

We should, as soon as possible, evaluate the latest research findings for their application in therapy. What we know now is certainly not enough, but it is a lot more than we knew 10 years ago. Dietary intervention must take fat into consideration. Fat calories are a measuring rod, not calories in general. Carbohydrates should be disregarded, and they should not now be considered in 'calorie mathematics'. Since this approach has been successful in many experimental studies it should also help patients. Behavioural therapy can support patients in establishing cognitive control (certainly of a flexible kind) in order to reduce fat intake. New foods that have a reduced fat content but provide similar sensual pleasure help, in a simple way, without great changes of behaviour. The image of foods containing carbohydrates must be made more attractive. If the opportunities for active exercise and for appropriate sports are used in the right way then it should be easier for obese people to become slimmer.

It can no longer be denied – although it can hardly be proved – that past methods of obesity therapy as well as the explanations given for weight gain contributed as psychogenetic factors to weight problems rather than resolving them. The practical application of the insights gained in obesity research is long overdue in order to avoid the repetition of earlier mistakes.

REFERENCES

Bouchard C, Tremblay A (1990). Genetic effects in human energy expenditure components. *International Journal of Obesity* **14** (Suppl. 1): 49–55.

Bouchard C, Tremblay A, Després J-P et al. (1990). The response to long-term overfeeding in identical twins. *New England Journal of Medicine* **322**: 1477–1482.

Brillat-Savarin J A (1971). *The Physiology of Taste* (translated from French by M F Fisher). Knopf, New York.

Brownell K D, Wadden T A (1986). Behaviour therapy for obesity: modern approaches and better results. In Brownell K D, Foreyt J P (eds) *Handbook of Eating Disorders*. New York: Basic Books, pp. 180–197.

Bruch H (1973). *Eating Disorders. Obesity, Anorexia Nervosa, and the Person Within*. New York: Basic Books.

Deutsche Gesellschaft für Ernährung (1992). *Ernährungsbericht 1992*. Druckerei Henrich, Frankfurt.

Ferster C B, Nurnberger J I, Levitt E E (1962). The control of eating. *Journal of Mathetics* **1**: 87–109.

Foreyt J P (ed.) (1977) *Behavioural Treatment of Obesity*. Pergammon Press Oxford.

Hauner H (1987). Fettgewebsverteilung und Adipositasrisiko. *Deutsche Medizinische Wochenschrift* **112**: 731–735.

Herman C P, Polivy J (1975). Anxiety, restraint and eating behaviour. *Journal of Abnormal Psychology* **84**: 666–672.

Herman C P, Polivy J (1984). A boundary model for the regulation of eating. In: Stunkard A J, Stellar E (eds) *Eating and its Disorders*. Raven Press, New York, pp. 141–156.

Kendall A, Levitsky D A, Strupp. B J, Lissner L (1991). Weight loss on a low fat diet, consequences of the imprecision of the control of food intake in humans. *American Journal of Clinical Nutrition* **53**: 1124–1129.

Keys A, Brozek J, Henschel A *et al*. (1950). *The Biology of Human Starvation*. University of Minnesota Press, Minneapolis.

Koehler K, Saß H (1984). *Diagnostisches und Statistisches Manual psychischer Störungen*, DSM III. Beltz, Weinheim.

Perri M G, Shapiro R M, Ludwig W W (1984). Maintenance strategies for the treatment of obesity. *Journal of Consulting and Clinical Psychology* **52**: 404–413.

Pudel V (1982). *Zur Psychogenese und Therapie der Adipositas*. Springer, Heidelberg.

Pudel V, Westenhöfer J (1989). *Fragebogen zum Eßverhalten: Handanweisung*. Hogrefe, Göttingen.

Pudel V, Westenhöfer J (1991). *Ernährungspsychologie*. Hogrefe, Göttingen.

Pudel V, Westenhöfer J (1992). Dietary and behavioural principles in the treatment of obesity. *International Monitor on Eating Patterns and Weight Control*, **1**(2): 2–7.

Pudel V, Metzdorff M, Oetting M (1975). Zur Persönlichkeit Adipöser in psychologischen Tests unter Berücksichtigung latent Fettsüchtiger. *Zeitschrift für Psychosomatische Medizin und Psychoanalyse* **21**: 345–361.

Russell G (1979). Bulimia nervosa: an ominous variant of anorexia nervosa. *Psychological Medicine* **9**: 429–448.

Schachter S (1968). Obesity and eating. *Science* **161**: 751–756.

Schachter S (1971). Some extraordinary facts about obese humans and rats. *American Psychologist* **26**: 129–144.

Schlundt D G, Hill J O, Pope-Cordle J *et al*. (1993). Randomised evaluation of a low fat *ad libitum* carbohydrate diet for weight reduction. *Journal of Obesity* **17**: 623–629.

Stunkard A J (1975). Presidential address – 1974: from explanation to action in psychosomatic medicine: the case of obesity. *Psychosomatic Medicine* **37**: 195–236.

Stunkard A J, Messick S (1985). The three-factor eating questionnaire to measure dietary restraint, disinhibition and hunger. *Journal of Psychosomatic Research* **29**: 71–83.

Vague J (1947). La differnciation sexuelle. Facteur déterminant des formes de l'obésité. *Press Med* **55**: 339–340.

Wallis H (1975). Psychosomatische Behandlungskonzepte der Adipositas im Kindesalter. *Monatsschrift für Kinderheilkunde* **123**: 264–272.

Westenhöfer J (1991a). *Gezügeltes Essen und Störbarkeit de Eßverhaltens.* Hogrefe, Göttingen.
Westenhöfer J (1991b). Dietary restraint and disinhibition: is restraint an homogenous construct? *Appetite* **16**: 45–55.
Westenhöfer J, Pudel V (1990). Einstellungen der deutschen Bevölkerung zum Essen. *Ernährungsumschau* **37**: 311–316.

CHAPTER 8

Realistic expectations of obesity treatments

Stephen Rössner

INTRODUCTION

In spite of numerous national campaigns and massive information to the general public, the mean body weight in Sweden, as well as in many other countries in the western world, has increased during the last decade (Kuskowska-Wolk and Rössner, 1990). Unfortunately, this undesirable development cannot be ascribed to the theoretically attractive explanation that fewer people smoke today (Boyle *et al.*, 1994; Wolk and Rössner, 1995). Smoking increases the basal metabolic rate by about 10% and smoking cessation generally results in a mean body weight increase of 3–4 kg (Rössner, 1986). In Sweden, the percentage of the population smoking has fallen during the 1980s from 32% to 27%, but this fall was not associated with the weight increase observed during the same time period. Similar findings were recently described in Australia (Boyle *et al.*, 1994).

Changes in physical activity also cannot explain the trend. Of particular concern, however, is the fact that physical activity seems to have become reduced and that obesity has become more prominent in children and adolescents (Sunnegård *et al.*, 1986; Gortmaker *et al.*, 1987).

NO NEW TREATMENT PRINCIPLES

Unfortunately, no dramatic breakthrough in obesity treatment has taken place or seems to be within immediate sight. The principal treatment modalities are basically still the same now as 20 years ago. The standard conservative treatment programmes still include diet, behavioural modification and exercise, although it should be admitted that these programmes

Weight Control
Edited by Richard Cottrell.
Published in 1995 by Chapman & Hall, London. ISBN 0 412 73600 4

have been better designed and now take into account the fact that obesity is a chronic condition that requires long-term treatment (Brownell and Jeffrey, 1987).

Surgical procedures may have undergone some technical improvements but are, in principle, still the same, resulting in restriction and, to a minor extent, in malabsorption, and will always be limited to a very small proportion of the obese population. Very low-calorie diets undergo minor changes in composition, energy content and regimens. They remain clearly very effective in short-term treatment but have not been shown to be a major factor in determining the long-term outcome of weight control over several years.

Drugs hold some promise for the future and new avenues are being explored, but the principal pharmacological intervention mechanism remains appetite suppression. Long-term drug treatment is rarely possible. Drugs probably have to be administered for several years to result in sustained weight reduction, and addiction has been a problem under some circumstances (Bray, 1993). In a number of countries, such as Sweden, the attitude of the regulating authorities to drug treatment of obesity has been so restrictive that no drug registered for weight reduction purposes is available on the market.

A PESSIMISTIC VIEW

This background description is a pessimistic way to look at the results of obesity treatment over the last decades, but is intended to emphasize that it is important that we have realistic expectations of what obesity treatment can achieve. If the ability to store excess energy as fat has been a survival mechanism during thousands of years of intermittent human starvation, it is perhaps surprising that most of us do not develop obesity, given the fact that today most people in the western world have access to food in excess of their needs. This development is rapidly becoming true also in eastern Europe. Since a change in energy balance theoretically seems so easy to achieve, both the general public and the medical profession have been led to believe that dramatic changes in body weight could be expected to occur in the same simple fashion as pneumonia can be readily cured by a few days' treatment with antibiotics. In the treatment of other diseases, such as rheumatism, psoriasis and AIDS, the results are even worse than in obesity treatment, but nobody questions the fact that vast resources are set aside by our societies in attempts to cope with these chronic, disabling and even lethal conditions.

As it has become obvious that long-term behavioural modification, leading to a sustained lower body weight, is difficult to achieve, the general population has given up the fight against overweight and obesity. The medical profession, realizing what little it has achieved in obesity treatment, has turned its back on the problem. Frank (1993), in a recent review, stated: 'The most common metabolic disease in the United States was treated with scorn, contempt and indifference'

WHY SO LITTLE SUCCESS?

In a critical review, Garner and Wooley (1991) have questioned the appropriateness of behavioural and dietary treatment of obesity in the light of what they considered overwhelming evidence that these treatment techniques were ineffective in producing lasting weight loss. They stated that:

- sustained weight loss for obese individuals does not equal improvement in health and longevity;
- a high, stable weight is safer than repeated weight fluctuations and that weight cycling may indeed even induce obesity;
- for many obese individuals, in particular moderately obese women, continuous dieting has untoward psychological effects, including depression, anxiety, social withdrawal and personality changes.

This paper has been much discussed. There is agreement about several of the facts mentioned by these authors, but that does not necessarily imply that obesity in principle should not be treated. Although it is possible that, in particular, women with moderate and benign obesity have little chance of becoming slim, other individuals, such as high-risk males with abdominal obesity, may benefit greatly from treatment. Improvements in the condition of patients with severe sleep apnoea syndrome, pains from weight-bearing joints, psychological disturbances or metabolic abnormalities can obviously be considerable, even from moderate weight loss. This means that individualization is a key element in decisions on obesity treatment strategies.

REALISTIC STRATEGIES

There are several reasons why it can be argued that obesity treatment has failed. One set of explanations relates to the three factors: the patient, the therapist and the environment, which all interact in determining the outcome of any weight loss programme.

The obese patient

In spite of all attempts, we still do not have any acceptable predictors of success in weight loss. There is as yet no questionnaire, no biopsy, no blood sample by which we can identify those patients in whom we can expect sustained weight loss with any clinically helpful reliability. This means that every day in the clinic we are actually wasting resources on patients for whom little can be done. Surgeons generally do not operate just to please patients, but base (or should base!) their decision to perform a surgical procedure on an evaluation which suggests that, on a risk–benefit basis, the patient has more to gain than to lose by the procedure. Quite often the obesity clinic tries to care for patients who have been referred by their physicians, or their anxious relatives, and have not primarily come of their own free will. Often for humanitarian reasons obese patients are accepted into programmes with which they have little likelihood of complying. They may wish to enter treatment at a period of their lives when many other complicating lifestyle changes will make it impossible to concentrate on the weight loss programme.

Another practical aspect concerns the ability of the weight loss clinic to address the particular problems of each patient. One such example relates to food intake over the day. Little clinical interest has been given to the fact that the food intake pattern over the day may determine the results of a weight loss programme. Most obese patients skip or have little breakfast, manage reasonably at lunchtime, but tend to eat more and more during the late afternoon and evening. Stunkard *et al.* (1955) identified a night eating problem, but since then little has been done to incorporate these observations into clinical practice. It is of little value to give advice about breakfast and lunch meals if the patient does not start to overeat until late in the evening. We have recently addressed the 'night eating syndrome' (NES) by analysing food intake during different hours of the day and by trying to identify factors typical of NES. Sixteen per cent of our obese patients showed a syndrome characterized by a predominant proportion of food energy intake being after 19.00 hours and either no sleep until after midnight or no breakfast. This eating pattern was virtually never seen in normal-weight subjects.

NES is an example of a common problem in obese patients that requires specific techniques to achieve success, just as binge eating disorder is another common feature of obesity. General advice will not help these patients, unless their specific eating problems are adequately addressed.

The therapist

Many different disciplines may be involved in the treatment of obesity, here for the sake of simplicity referred to as 'therapists'. Murphree (1994) has summarized the situation when one of these actors, the family physician, meets the obese patient. She clearly emphasizes that theoretically adequate recommendations from the therapist will not result in sustained weight loss in the patients, unless the physician manages to identify what conditions will really make the patient actually change behaviour. Her patients were reluctant to change their eating habits ('diets not appetizing') or to increase the amount of exercise undertaken ('time-consuming, boring, painful') and did not want to visit a physician or dietitian on their own ('I don't want to be told to eat salad and drink water'). Murphree concluded that to achieve any success in such patients it is important to develop programmes that include:

- group therapy;
- 'group exercise';
- new approaches to transport and child care issues;
- instruction in modification of currently used recipes;
- dietary modification addressing food taste and texture, not only energy content.

These observations, derived from focus group meetings, highlight the importance of designing realistic weight loss programmes. Elegant and theoretically appropriate hypocaloric regimens will not result in weight loss if the obese patient cannot find a babysitter while attending the weight loss sessions!

The environment

Not only the colleagues of Frank (1993) but also the environment of the obese patient as a whole demonstrate a negative attitude towards obesity. Treatment resources for obesity are not made generally available in countries such as Sweden, although there is a national medical health care system.

Obesity creates a stigma even in childhood. Harris and Smith (1983) found by showing pictures of individuals of varying shape that normal-weight children were seen as happier, smarter, better looking, less lonely and having more friends than those who were overweight. This stigmatization will follow obese patients into their adult lives, e.g. obese job applicants are viewed negatively (Rothblum *et al.*, 1988; Klesges *et al.*, 1990).

To a great extent these negative attitudes of society towards obesity are mediated by the mass media. On the one hand, modern television provides the public with a 'television diet' that is certainly not consistent with the general principles of sound nutrition (Rössner, 1990). On the other hand, the actors on the television screen are hardly ever overweight. In the study by Kaufmann (1980) only 15% of the men and 8% of the women were represented as overweight or obese, and overweight children or teenagers were hardly ever shown on TV. Thus, the overemphasis on leanness, as reflected in the selection of attractive women in beauty contests, as well as the general message from the powerful television industry, will help to underscore the impression that leanness is associated with success and that overweight and obesity are associated with failure.

The discrimination against overweight and obesity in several educational, occupational, racial, ethnic and geographical areas, and in society, seems the more unjustified as it has become clear that overweight individuals do not show more psychological disturbances than are found in the general population. Obese patients seen for medical or surgical procedures do not exhibit more psychopathology than do non-obese patients (Wadden and Stunkard, 1985).Thus some of the most severe complications of obesity are in fact consequences of the contemptuous attitude of society. It remains important to emphasize that hardly any individual who has developed overweight and obesity set out in life to strive for an excess of body weight.

THE DEFINITION OF SUCCESS

The patient, the therapist and the environment may hold unrealistic expectations of what constitutes failure and success in the treatment of obesity. Atkinson (1993) has recently proposed standards for judging the success of a treatment programme. One approach concerns the evaluation of body weight changes, expressed in kilograms, percentage of excess body weight, BMI, etc. Other ways to judge success are to evaluate the maintenance of improvement over time, the attrition rate of a given programme and the reduction in complications and the need for obesity-associated treatments. Since successes cannot always be defined in simple terms, a new approach using 'pattern analysis' is of interest (Holman *et al.*, 1994). By this technique a pattern of interest can be defined a priori and the proportion of patients in different treatment programmes attaining the given pattern can be compared. This makes it possible to compare various factors associated with weight reduction, such as weight loss, body mass composition or change in risk factors, and permits an objective summary and statistical data analysis. In a similar way we recently analysed lifestyle factors affecting body weight development after pregnancy. Figure 8.1 demonstrates the weight development in women 1 year after delivery with different changes in snack frequency before, during and after pregnancy (Öhlin and Rössner, 1994).

AN OPTIMISTIC VIEW

Several important reasons why obesity treatment is often unsuccessful have been summarized here. It seems important, however, to include also some practical suggestions to overcome the obstacles. It is important to have a long-term perspective and not to expect dramatic changes in attitudes to body weight and lifestyle.

Weight loss programmes have effects on subjects other than the patients in treatment. We recently interviewed patients in our weight loss programme and found that, in addition to the 11.9 ± 9.0 kg lost by 85 obese

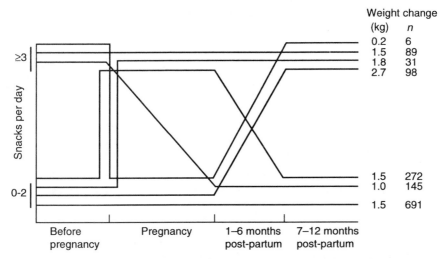

Figure 8.1 Effect of snacking frequency on weight changes during pregnancy and post-partum. Data from Ohlin and Rössner (1994).

patients, 37 of their close relatives had lost a mean of 6.1 ± 4.2 kg (Franson and Rössner, 1994).

Whereas most media experts agree that the time of mass information is overdue, simple, cheap activities may be incorporated into everyday life, helping individuals to make choices that will improve their chances of controlling body weight. Brownell *et al.* (1980) doubled the use of stairs in a shopping mall just by placing a colourful sign encouraging the use of stairs instead of the escalator. By placing a similar sign in a Stockholm subway exit we reduced the proportion of people using escalator from 98% to 85%.

The Stockholm City Theatre has for several years been showing a lunch performance including a healthy lunch meal and a comical, sympathetic education play on body weight, lifestyle and eating behaviour. This play has also been broadcast on Swedish prime-time television and has stimulated media interest in sound advice for obese subjects.

In Australia the high-risk group of obese men has been addressed with a programme called *Gutbusters* 'for the men with the guts to give it a go!'. Similarly, in Stockholm we have addressed obese high-risk men in the Gustaf programme ('Gustaf' being the Swedish translation of Garfield, the fat cat). Preliminary results are promising.

In her thesis, Kanström (1994) demonstrated that by manipulating the order of the menus of 32 restaurants, placing the healthiest dish on the top of the list, 6% of the customers could be made to chose a healthier alternative.

These examples demonstrate that using creativity and imagination simple steps can be taken that by no means solve the problem but may help to reduce the long-term risk of failure.

REFERENCES

Atkinson R L (1993). Proposed standards for judging the success of the treatment of obesity. *Annals of Internal Medicine* **119**: 677–680.

Boyle C A, Dobson A J, Egger G, Magnus P (1994). Can the increasing weight of Australians be explained by the decreasing prevalence of cigarette smoking? *International Journal of Obesity* **18**: 55–60.

Bray G A (1993). Use and abuse of appetite-suppressant drugs in the treatment of obesity. *Annals of Internal Medicine* **119**: 707–713.

Brownell K, Jeffery R (1987). Improving long term weight loss: pushing the limits of treatment. *Behavioural Therapy* **18**: 353–362.

Brownell K D, Stunkard A J, Albaum J M (1980). Evaluation and modification of exercise patterns in the natural environment. *American Journal of Psychiatry* **137**: 1540–1545.

Frank A (1993). Futility and avoidance. Medical professionals in the treatment of obesity. *JAMA* **269**: 2132–2133.

Franson K, Rössner S (1994). Effects of weight reduction programmes on close family members. *International Journal of Obesity* **18** (in press).

Garner M D, Wooley C S (1991). Confronting the failure of behavioural and dietary treatments for obesity. *Clinical Psychology Review* **11**: 729–780.

Gortmaker S L, Dietwz W H, Sobol A M, Wehler C A (1987). Increasing paediatric obesity in the United States. *American Journal of Diseases in Children* **141**: 535–540.

Harris M B, Smith S D (1983). The relationships of age, sex, ethnicity and weight to stereotypes of obesity and self perception. *International Journal of Obesity* **17**: 361–371.

Holman S L, Goldstein D L, Enas G G (1994). Pattern analysis method for assessing successful weight reduction. *International Journal of Obesity* **18**: 281–285.

Kanström L (1994). Community-based methods and tools to promote dietary changes: some experiences from the Stockholm Cancer Prevention Programme. Thesis, Karolinska Institute, Stockholm.

Kauffman L (1980). Prime-time nutrition. *Journal of Community Health* **30**: 37–46.

Klesges R C, Klem M L, Hanson C L et al. (1990). The effects of applicant's health status and qualifications on simulated hiring decisions. *International Journal of Obesity* **14**: 527–535.

Kuskowska-Wolk A, Rössner S (1990). Prevalence of obesity in Sweden. *Journal of Internal Medicine* **227**: 241–246.

Murphree D (1994). Patient attitude toward physician treatment of obesity. *J Fam Pract* **38**: 45–48.

Öhlin A, Rössner S (1994). Trends in eating patterns, physical activity and socio-demographic factors in relation to postpartum body weight development. *British Journal of Nutrition* **71**: 457–470.

Rössner S (1986). Cessation of cigarette smoking and body weight increase (editorial). *Acta Medica Scandinavica* **219**: 1–2.

Rössner S (1990). Television viewing, life style and obesity. *Journal of Internal Medicine* **229**: 301–302.

Rothblum E D, Miller C T, Garbutt B (1988). Stereotypes of obese female job applicants. *International Journal of Eating Disorders* **7**: 277–283.

Stunkard A J, Grace J W, Wolff H G (1955). The night eating syndrome. *Am J Med* **19**: 78–86.

Sunnegård J, Bratteby L E, Hagman U, Samuelson G, Sjölin S (1986). Physical activity in relation to energy intake and body fat in 8 and 13 year-old children in Sweden. *Acta Paediatrica Scandinavica* **75**: 955–963.

Wadden T A, Stunkard A J (1985). Social and psychological consequences of obesity. *Annals of Internal Medicine* **103**: 1062–1067.
Wolk A, Rössner S (1995). Effects of smoking and physical activity on body weight development in Sweden. *Journal of Internal Medicine* **235**: 287–291.

CHAPTER 9

Health professional approach to weight control

Xavier Formiguera

Until recently, most people, including many health professionals, considered obesity in a frivolous manner, as if it were merely an aesthetic problem. But obesity is much more than a simple question of good looks, and today there is no doubt that obesity, especially 'central-type' obesity, is a health problem, and in many developed countries, constitutes a public health problem.

There are two main reasons for this. First, there is a strong association with morbidity and mortality. Numerous epidemiological studies, especially prospective studies with long-term follow-up, such as the Framingham Study (Hubert *et al.*, 1983), the study of men born in 1913 (Larsson *et al.*, 1984), the San Antonio Heart Study (Golay *et al.*, 1988) and others, clearly demonstrate strong associations between the degree of obesity and the occurrence of diseases of metabolic or cardiovascular origin.

Data from the Framingham Study illustrate the relationship between obesity, expressed in terms of relative weight according to the Metropolitan Life Insurance Company tables of desirable weight, and the occurrence of ischaemic heart attack: the higher the weight, the greater the probability of having a heart attack.

Table 9.1, based on the data from NAHNES II (Briefel, 1994), demonstrates a clear relationship between obesity, diabetes and arterial hypertension. Note that diabetes and arterial hypertension are twice as prevalent in obese people as in those not obese. This positive relationship is even stronger in black people.

In considering the adverse effects of obesity on health status it is necessary to take into account not only BMI but also, and perhaps more importantly, the pattern of body fat distribution.

Weight Control
Edited by Richard Cottrell.
Published in 1995 by Chapman & Hall, London. ISBN 0 412 73600 4

Table 9.1 Risk factor prevalence by race and obesity (yes or no) in USA, 1976–80

	White men		White women		Black men		Black women	
	Yes	No	Yes	No	Yes	No	Yes	No
Hypercholesterolaemia	31	23	40	26	33	20	33	18
Hypertension	56	27	51	19	63	32	62	26
Hypercholesterolaemia and hypertension	20	9	24	9	25	9	22	10
Type II diabetes mellitus	4	2	7	2	8	2	9	2

From studies by Vague (1947, 1956), we know that there are two main types of obesity that differ in the regional distribution of fat deposits in the body. Björntorp (1993) and others (e.g. Seidell *et al.*, 1989) started to establish a clear relationship between central-type obesity and an increased occurrence of metabolic and cardiovascular disease. It is now clear that central obesity constitutes an independent risk factor for cardiovascular diseases.

The second reason for considering obesity a public health problem is because of its high prevalence in the so-called 'developed countries'.

Table 9.2 is a meta-analysis of a number of epidemiological studies carried out in different countries. According to Garrow's (1981) classification of obesity it can be seen that grade I obesity is more prevalent among men, whereas the prevalence of grade II and III obesity is higher in women. As shown here, the overall prevalence of grade II and III obesity (that is when BMI is over 30 kg m^{-2}), is over 12% in some populations, which is a prevalence approximately three times higher than that observed for diabetes.

Table 9.2 Prevalence of obesity

Country	Age (years)	Overweight (%)		Obesity (%)	
		Men	Women	Men	Women
UK	16–55	34	24	6	8
Australia	25–64	34	24	7	7
Switzerland	16–84	35	26	7	8
USA	20–74	34	24	12	12
Italy	20–60	41	26	12	14

Overweight: BMI = 25–30; obesity: BMI > 30.

So, when the question is 'To treat or not to treat obesity?', my answer is clearly 'yes'.

But weight control is not easy, and often, the long-term results of intervention are poor and discouraging. Only a small percentage of patients achieve an 'ideal weight' for their lifetime.

There are a number of reasons for this. The first is that obesity has a multifactorial origin. Genetic factors play an important role, conferring the possibility of becoming obese. Nevertheless, genetic factors alone do not explain fully what usually occurs in clinical practice. Environmental factors are also essential to the development of obesity. Thus, it is generally accepted that, one or more environmental factors, acting on a genetically obesity-prone individual, enable the expression of the disease. Therefore, we can say that genetics confers the possibility of becoming obese, whereas the environment determines the moment of appearance and the magnitude of the disease.

Another reason that makes it difficult to achieve good long-term results is the chronic character of the disease that makes it mandatory that it is treated for life. Everybody is able to be a hero for a short period of time, but few are capable of permanently changing their lifestyle (eating habits, exercise, etc.). Nowadays this is especially difficult because almost everybody makes deals, celebrates victories and talks about their troubles around the dining table.

The third factor that hinders obesity treatment is that, usually, therapeutic measures are more bothersome than the disease itself. Obesity is painless, and in the first years, when the patient is young, the disease is generally well tolerated. In these early stages, when complications have not yet appeared, it is very difficult to convince the patient to start a weight control programme.

Finally, as obesity is a multifactorial disease, treatment must also consider different aspects, otherwise the use of single therapeutic measures will lead to poor and inconsistent results in almost all cases.

Taking into account all of these considerations, let us review which are the main weapons we have to combat obesity and how to use them.

Since obesity is a result of an imbalance between energy income and energy expenditure, the global approach to its treatment must be directed to correct this imbalance, trying both to reduce energy intake and to increase energy expenditure.

HYPOCALORIC DIET

The key to weight control is the hypocaloric diet. The degree of calorie restriction must be adapted, when possible, to individual daily energy requirements.

We are not concerned here with constructing a hypocaloric diet, but in my opinion every diet must:

- provide the minimal daily requirements of macro- and micronutrients;
- respect gastronomic preferences;
- take into account unchangeable conditions (age, race, sex, pregnancy, etc.);
- adapt to mode of unemployment and work schedule;
- be pleasant and palatable, maintaining the hedonistic values of food;
- avoid absolute prohibitions.

The more varied the diet, the better compliance will be.

In our opinion there are no bad foods, but what is wrong is the abuse of some foods. We firmly believe that no food is to be prohibited, but obviously reduction of some energy-dense foods, such as fat, is necessary. Moderate amounts of sugar should be permitted since total prohibitions often induce cravings that may worsen an underlying compulsive or bulimic-like eating behaviour.

Dietary counselling should be focused primarily on achieving long-term changes in eating habits rather than on losing a great amount of weight. Moderately restrictive mixed diets should result in a loss of 0.5 kg per week, i.e. 26 kg per year, which is easier to achieve.

EXERCISE

The role of exercise in obesity treatment is controversial. Theoretically, exercise will result in a further increase in energy expenditure, which should contribute to increase weight loss. However, in practice, weight loss is almost always less than expected. In fact, most studies on the role of exercise alone in obesity treatment have failed to demonstrate significant weight reductions. Furthermore, exercise increases appetite, which may hinder diet compliance.

All of these observations do not invalidate the benefits of exercise in obese patients. Exercise can modify body composition, enhancing muscular mass, and therefore preventing the fall in resting metabolic rate (RMR) that usually accompanies a loss of fat mass.

As can be seen in Table 9.3, different studies find similar results showing that loss of weight results in a significant reduction in RMR measured by indirect calorimetry. This fall in RMR is presumably due to the decrease in FFM. Thus, the exercise-induced increase in muscle mass can contribute to the avoidance of a decrease in RMR that would otherwise invariably occur.

But perhaps the most interesting use of exercise is in the weight maintenance phase. In Figure 9.1, obtained from the data of Pavlou *et al.* (1989), a significant difference in weight regain is seen between patients treated with a balanced hypocaloric diet alone and those treated with the same diet combined with a physical exercise programme. Therefore,

Table 9.3 RMR before (RMR 1) and after (RMR 2) weight loss

Reference		Weight loss (kg)	RMR 1 (kcal 24 h^{-1})	RMR 2 (kcal 24 h^{-1})
Bessard	1983	11.7	1661	1423
Schutz	1984	13.4	2275	1843
Welle	1984	10.8	1552	1380
Formiguera	1988	13.8	1607	1572

exercise seems to have an interesting effect on the prevention of weight relapse, especially in association with behavioural programmes.

The beneficial affects of exercise other than weight control include reduction in blood pressure, improvements in lipid profile, helping to increase high-density lipoprotein (HDL)-cholesterol and reducing low-density lipoprotein (LDL)-cholesterol and triglyceride levels and improvement in glucose metabolism through an increase in insulin sensitivity.

A further issue is the intensity of exercise. Much evidence suggests that moderate exercise, such as regular walking, is more beneficial for obese persons than intense exercise.

PHARMACOTHERAPY

There are a number of different drugs that can be used to treat obesity. They can be classified in different groups according to their mode of action.

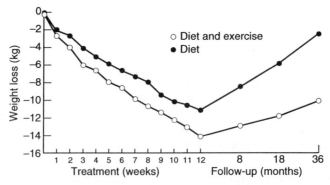

Figure 9.1 Effect of exercise on weight loss. ●, Diet; ○, diet + exercise. Data from Pavlou *et al.* (1989) Exercise as an adjunct to weight loss and maintenance in moderately obese subjects, *American Journal of Clinical Nutrition*, **49**, 1115–1123, © *American Journal of Clinical Nutrition*, American Society for Clinical Nutrition, reproduced with permission.

Anorexigens

Anorectic drugs suppress appetite and can play a useful role in any overall weight control programme. Reducing appetite or enhancing satiety makes it easier to pursue a hypocaloric diet. They should always be used in conjunction with diet and other therapeutic measures, never alone.

Catecholaminergic drugs

Catecholaminergic compounds, such as diethylpropion, suppress appetite, increasing the hypothalamic levels of adrenaline and noradrenaline, thus stimulating β_2-adrenoreceptors. They have side-effects derived from this β_2 stimulation that can lead to tachycardia, hypertension, nervousness, tremor, etc., and they are potentially addictive.

Serotoninergic drugs

Serotoninergic drugs have been introduced more recently. Dexfenfluramine, the dextrorotatory stereoisomer of fenfluramine, increases hypothalamic serotonin action in two ways: increasing serotonin release and decreasing its reuptake in serotoninergic synapsis.

Fluoxetine acts mainly by blocking serotonin reuptake.

The rise in hypothalamic serotonin has been demonstrated to have a macronutrient selection effect in animals. Direct injection of serotonin into the hypothalamic nucleus causes changes in rat macronutrient selection. When serotonin is injected in the paraventricular nucleus a decrease in carbohydrate intake is observed, while the appetite for proteins is enhanced. A similar macronutrient selection pattern is seen when serotonin is injected into the ventromedial nucleus. In the suprachiasmatic nucleus a global reduction in macronutrient intake is observed.

This serotonin-induced macronutrient selection, clearly demonstrated in rats, has been also observed in humans. Treatment with dexfenfluramine reduces daily caloric intake, decreasing the intake of carbohydrates with no effect on protein ingestion.

Dexfenfluramine seems to be free of the tolerance effect. The study by Guy Grand *et al.* (1989) demonstrated that there is no loss of effectiveness during the 1 year of treatment. The amount of weight lost was significantly greater in a dexfenfluramine group than in a placebo group.

Fluoxetine, the other serotoninergic compound, is an antidepressant that acts by blocking serotonin reuptake. Like the other compounds in the group, it reduces food intake and decreases appetite for carbohydrates. It is especially useful in depressed obese patients, in carbohydrate cravers and in those with binge eating disorder together, of course, with psychotherapy support.

Thermogenic drugs

Thermogenic drugs are now under investigation. They act through β_3-adrenergic receptors, increasing thermogenesis. Weight-reducing effects are well demonstrated in animals. So far there have been few studies in humans, but results are encouraging. β_3 selectivity is not absolute and mild side-effects on the cardiovascular system are usually observed. Further studies are projected by pharmaceutical companies, but, as yet, these drugs should be considered only on a research basis.

The main goals of obesity treatment are to lose weight and to avoid weight regain. The best treatment of obesity must be considered for each individual. Better results will be obtained if a hypocaloric diet, moderate daily exercise and behavioural therapy, are used simultaneously as a basis for a change in lifestyle. The rational use of pharmacotherapy will, in many cases, help to achieve these goals.

In some cases patients fail to adhere to such a conventional weight control programme for a number of reasons. If the patient is morbidly obese or has an obesity-related disease, very low-calorie diets (VLCDs) may be helpful to achieve weight loss.

Indications for the use of VLCDs are the following:

- morbid obesity;
- presence of obesity-related diseases;
- failure of previous attempts to lose weight.

If used properly, they are safe and effective, but severe myocardial disease or pregnancy constitutes a formal contraindication to their use.

VERY LOW-CALORIE DIETS

In a prospective study (Formiguera *et al.*, 1991) 62 morbidly obese patients were treated with a VLCD containing 400 kcal per day for 4 weeks. The tolerance was good and the results were as follows. The total amount of weight lost was 15 kg, of which 9 kg was FM and 6 kg was FFM. BMI decreased from 43.5 to 34.7 kg m^{-2}.

Nitrogen balance was negative throughout the study but with a tendency to normalize during the last few days.

SURGERY

Finally, surgical procedures should be considered if all previous attempts have failed to achieve weight loss in patients with morbid obesity or in those with grade II obesity or above who have related diseases susceptible to improvement if weight is reduced significantly (for example sleep apnoea syndrome, type II diabetes mellitus).

In our experience (Formiguera *et al.*, 1989) vertical band gastroplasty (VBG) produces good weight loss with few side-effects. The goal of the technique is to reduce gastric capacity in order to achieve earlier satiety and delayed gastric emptying.

The stomach is perforated approximately 7 cm from the oesophago-gastric union and 3 cm inside the minor curvature. Both gastric walls are perforated and stapled with a circular suture by means of an end-to-end intestinal suture device. Then, a Goretex or Teflon ribbon is passed through the orifice, both ends being sutured. The function of this band is to avoid the excessive opening of the stoma and to control gastric pouch emptying. Finally, with a stapler device a suture from the orifice to the gastric fundus is made, creating a 'reservoir' of 25–30 cm^3 capacity.

The procedure is generally well tolerated. The main complications arise from the failure of the vertical stapled suture in about 20% of cases.

Since 1988 my group has been studying 130 patients who have been treated with VBG for morbid obesity. There are 96 females and 34 males with an average age of 34 ± 9.8 years and a BMI of 49.8 kg m^{-2}. The initial waist–hip ratio (WHR) was 0.93 ± 0.3 for females and 1.07 for males. All of them fulfil the criteria for inclusion in our Obesity Surgical Treatment Programme and have undergone a VBG using Mason's technique. Assessments were made before the surgical procedure and then at 3, 6 and 12 months and yearly following surgery. In these controls we evaluated changes in anthropometric parameters (weight, overweight, BMI and WHR) and the variations in lipidic profile, plasma glucose values and transaminases (in our opinion the best indicator of hepatic steatosis, as we previously reported in a communication at the 3rd European Congress on Obesity in Nice).

Figure 9.2 shows the pattern of weight loss during the 3 years after VBG. As usual, weight shows a rapid decrease in the first 6 months followed by a slower fall and then by a third phase of stabilization that in our patients took place between 12 and 18 months.

BMI also decreased and followed a three-step curve from an initial value of 49.8 kg m^{-2} to 31.9 kg m^{-2} in the first 12 months, maintaining a similar level thereafter.

Figure 9.3 shows the variations we have found in the regional pattern of fat distribution. Our definition of central-type obesity is a WHR over 0.85 in women and over 1 in men. As shown in the figure, WHR clearly decreased in men from a baseline value of 1.07 and was maintained at < 1 over the whole 3-year follow-up. In contrast, in women, the WHR did not change significantly and remained above 0.85 throughout the follow-up period.

The lipid profile exhibits significant changes. Total cholesterol did not vary during follow-up, but there was a slight decrease in LDL-cholesterol level, a significant increase in HDL-cholesterol and a marked reduction in triglyceride values (Figure 9.4).

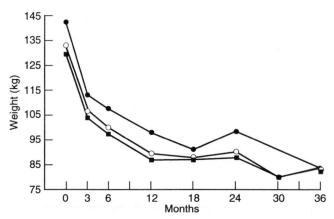

Figure 9.2   Changes in weight following vertical banded gastroplasty.
○, Women; ●, men; ■ total.

Transaminases also show a rapid decline in the first 6 months, indicating an improvement in hepatic steatosis; levels thereafter remained normal.

Finally, in the 21 type II diabetic patients studied (16% of all patients) the fasting plasma glucose values fell dramatically in the first 3 months, reaching near-normal values after 12 months. This enabled us to reduce substantially or even eliminate oral hypoglycaemic therapy in all cases.

Our findings can be summarized as follows.

- The weight loss achieved after VBG in our 130 patients was considerable and was maintained over a 3-year follow-up period.
- This level of weight loss (46 kg) was associated with favourable and sustained modifications in all the cardiovascular risk factors related to obesity that were examined.
- In type II diabetic patients plasma glucose concentrations fell significantly and remained at normal levels throughout the follow-up period. This was, in fact, the result of a decrease in insulin resistance.

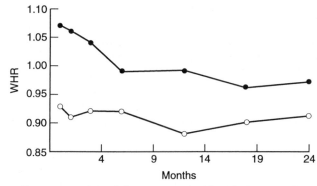

Figure 9.3   Changes in WHR following vertical banded gastroplasy. ○, Women ($n = 41$); ●, men ($n = 16$).

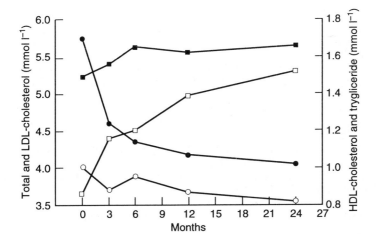

Figure 9.4   Changes in lipid profile following vertical banded gastroplasty.
■, Total cholesterol; □, HDL-cholesterol; ●, triglyceride; ○, LDL-cholesterol.

- The weight loss induced by VBG was thus able to improve the 'metabolic syndrome'.
- In men, VBG induced a gradual change in the body fat distribution from a 'central' type to a less aggressive intermediate pattern. WHR was not substantially altered in women.
- There was also an important improvement in hepatic steatosis manifested by the normalization of plasma transaminase values.

REFERENCES

Björntorp P (1992). Regional obesity. In: Björntorp P, Brodoff B N (eds) *Obesity*. J B Lippincott, Philadelphia, pp. 579–586.

Briefel R R (1994) Assessment of the US diet in national nutrition surveys: national collaborative efforts and NHANES. *American Journal of Clinical Nutrition* **59** (Suppl), 1645–1675.

Formiguera X, Alastrué A, Rull M *et al.* (1989). Anthropometric changes in patients with morbid obesity undergoing vertical banded gastroplasty: results of one year follow-up. *International Journal of Obesity* **13** (Suppl. 1): 207.

Formiguera X, Barbany M, Carrillo M, Galan A, Herrero P, Foz M (1991). Modificaciones antropométricas y balance de nitrógeno en pacientes con obesidad mórbida tratados con una dieta baja en calorías. *Med Clin* **96**: 401–404.

Golay A, Felber J P, Jéquier E, DeFronzo R A, Ferranini E (1988). Metabolic basis of obesity and non-insulin-dependent diabetes. *Diab Metab Rev* **4**: 727–747.

Garrow J S (1981) *Treat Obesity Seriously*. Churchill Livingstone, London.

Guy Grand B, Crepaldi G, Lefebvre P *et al.* (1989). International trial of long-term dexfenfluramine in obesity. *Lancet* **ii**: 1142–1144.

Hubert H B, Feinleib M, McNamara P M *et al.* (1983). Obesity as an independent risk factor for cardiovascular disease. A 26-year follow-up of participants in the Framingham Heart Study. *Circulation* **67**: 968.

Larsson B, Svardsudd K, Welin L, Wilhelmsen L *et al.* (1984). Abdominal adipose tissue distribution, obesity and risk of cardiovascular disease and death: 13-year follow-up of participants in the study of men born in 1913. *British Medical Journal* **288**: 1401–1404.

Pavlou K N, Krey S, Steffe W P (1989). Exercise as an adjunct to weight loss and maintenance in moderately obese subjects. *American Journal of Clinical Nutrition* **49**: 1115–1123.

Seidell J C, Björntorp P, Sjöström L, Sannerstedt R *et al.* (1989). Regional distribution of muscle and fat mass in men: new insight into the risk of abdominal obesity using computed tomography. *International Journal of Obesity* **13**: 289–303.

The 3rd European Congress on Obesity, Nice, 1992, published as *Obesity in Europe 1991*, John Libbey, London, 1992.

Vague J (1947). La differenciation sexuelle: factor determinant des formes de l'obesité. *Press Med* **55**: 339–340.

Vague J (1956). The degree of masculine differentiation of obesities: a factor determining predisposition to diabetes, atherosclerosis, gout and uric calculous disease. *American Journal of Clinical Nutrition* **4**: 20–34.

Index